WHAT EVERY PIANIST
NEEDS TO KNOW ABOUT THE BODY

WHAT EVERY PIANIST NEEDS TO KNOW ABOUT THE BODY

A manual for players of keyboard instruments

PIANO • ORGAN • DIGITAL KEYBOARD • HARPSICHORD • CLAVICHORD

By Thomas Mark

•

with

Supplementary Material for Organists

By Roberta Gary and Thom Miles

•

Based on

WHAT EVERY MUSICIAN NEEDS TO KNOW ABOUT THE BODY

By Barbara Conable

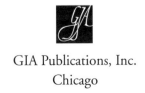

GIA Publications, Inc.

Chicago

G-5883
© 2003 GIA Publications, Inc.
7404 S. Mason Ave., Chicago, IL 60638
www.giamusic.com
ISBN: 1-57999-206-4

Book layout and back cover design: Kendra Hume Design
Front cover: Lael Cyr
Artwork: Benjamin Conable, from *What Every Musician Needs to Know about the Body,* used by permission. Artwork on pp. 21, 37, 60, 90, 91, 99, 102, 104, 106, 110, 111, 113, 114, and 116 is the work of Marco Gonzales. Artwork on p. 35 is the work of Barbara Conable and William Conable.

Excerpts from an early version of Chapter 9 appeared in *The Oregon Musician,* Spring, 1999.

Printed in the United States of America

For Susan

Table of Contents

꒰

PREFACE

The text of this book is by Thomas Mark. The concept of the body map and the power of Body Mapping in improving movement and curing injury among musicians were the joint discovery of Barbara Conable and William Conable. In her book, *What Every Musician Needs to Know about the Body*, Barbara Conable presented the basic information required by musicians for developing an accurate and adequate body map. This book presents the same information in somewhat different form, with much more detailed verbal description, expanding and adapting it for players of keyboard instruments. Most of the illustrations come from *What Every Musician Needs to Know about the Body* and are the work of Benjamin Conable. Additional illustrations are the work of Marco Gonzales. The portions of the book addressed specifically to the needs of organists are the work of Roberta Gary and Thom Miles.

This book is for players of all keyboard instruments: piano, organ, harpsichord, clavichord, and digital keyboard. All players of keyboard instruments need the information offered here and should adapt and apply it to their particular instruments. The arm and hand have the same structure and the same possibilities of movement whether someone is playing piano, organ, or something else. Players who understand the structure can generate free, efficient movement on whatever instrument is being played. Similarly, because keyboard instruments are played sitting down, players of keyboard instruments need to understand what it means to sit in balance. Organists need to know all this and more, since their instrument poses some demands different from other keyboard instruments. Therefore, this book includes special sections for organists.

Although the information in this book is for all players of keyboard instruments, "player of a keyboard instrument" is a cumbersome phrase. For that reason, and because I am a pianist myself, I generally use the word "pianist" in the text. Most players of keyboard instruments other than piano do also play the piano, so I hope that all readers will feel that the word "pianist" includes them.

This book is intended to help pianists develop a heightened sense of their own structure and movement at the piano. But for most people, actual demonstration can clarify the subject far more effectively than mere verbal description. Therefore, a video, also entitled *What Every Pianist Needs to Know about the Body,* is available from GIA Publications (VHS-566). In it, I demonstrate standing and sitting in balance, motions of the hand and arm, and other topics from the book, both at the piano and away from it. Most readers will find the video a worthwhile supplement to the book.

I have benefited from criticism and comments from colleagues Jane Buttars, Amy Likar, Molly Sloter, Jeanne Weisman, and Kathryn Woodard. Anita King read several drafts of the manuscript and her comments have been especially thoughtful, comprehensive, and constructive. My greatest debt is to Barbara Conable, who gave assistance and insight at every stage of preparation.

Thomas Mark

INTRODUCTION

A few years ago I was practicing the Sonata in A major, K. 113, by Scarlatti, which contains rapid wide leaps for the left hand. I noticed that if I sat up "straight" I missed fewer of the leaps. Intrigued, I went to see an expert in posture and movement who gave me some exercises intended to improve my posture. Later, I became acquainted with the work of Barbara Conable, and came to understand that awareness and coordination of the entire body influence—indeed, they determine—the quality and safety of our piano playing. What I learned has transformed my playing and teaching.

This is not a book about piano technique. I shall say little about how to play arpeggios and nothing about fingering the B-flat major scale in thirds. Nor is it a book about the Alexander Technique, although anyone familiar with F. M. Alexander's work will recognize that the book builds on his insights, in particular his recognition that the way we use our bodies makes a huge difference to how well we perform specific tasks. Instead, I offer anatomical facts that may seem, at first, to be irrelevant to playing the piano.

The information in this book will be new to many pianists, but when properly assimilated it brings about improved bodily awareness, a better quality of movement, and better piano playing. Indeed, it can transform a person's playing. It does not take the place of technique. Rather, it is what permits technique to function. Even a good technique, with efficient use of the fingers, hands, and forearms, can yield playing that sounds wooden and is insecure if the proper involvement and support of the rest of the body is lacking.

The information is vital for another reason also: it enables us to avoid and recover from injury. Nowadays, there is a near epidemic of musicians' injuries, and many musicians who do not consider themselves injured still experience fatigue and limitation. I know of no reliable way to estimate the proportion of professional musicians who suffer injury, but some people say it is over fifty percent, and higher among pianists. The precise figure is not important; what is important is that injury is very common.

Many pianists, once injured, become deeply discouraged because no one seems able to help them. This is tragic because injury is avoidable and curable. In almost all cases, pianists who obtain accurate information and proper instruction can recover completely from injury. Unfortunately, the knowledge needed to avoid injury and restore injured pianists to health is not part of most pianists' training. This book is intended to meet the need.

Because injuries are so common I do consistently point out their causes. But no one should suppose that this emphasis on avoiding injury means that the book is valuable only to injured pianists. Every pianist, injured or not, will benefit from the information offered here. Teachers have a special responsibility to acquire it, since only by mastering it and making it part of their teaching can they help students reach their full potential without risk of pain and injury.

This is a book about how we move our bodies to play the piano.

Thomas Mark

INTRODUCTION FOR ORGANISTS

As a student in Montreal in the early 1970s I was afforded the luxury of practicing the organ five or six hours a day. I continued this habit when I moved to Cincinnati a few years later to begin work at the College-Conservatory of Music. What I perceived to be bad luck intervened, however, and within a year of beginning my studies in Cincinnati I developed severe tendonitis in my right hand and wrist. A few weeks later the pain manifested itself in my left hand as well. Thus began an almost decade-long search for relief from pain, followed at last by a return to normal playing and practicing. I consulted hand specialists, chiropractors, and yoga instructors. Nothing worked until in the early 1980s I had the good fortune of meeting Barbara Conable. She watched me play for a few minutes, then announced, "We have work to do." The work we did over time returned my hands and arms to pain-free playing. This was accomplished by retraining my movements at the organ. Painful playing is now part of my past, and I have no fear of the pain returning. I also play more freely and musically. What more could one ask?

The information in this book is vital for organists as well as pianists. Though piano and organ techniques differ in many ways, the proper use of the body does not change as one moves from one instrument to the other. Nor do differing technical or musical approaches to organ playing change the underlying principles of proper use of the body. Organists, please read carefully and take to heart all of the information directed to pianists. As you read you will also find material directed specifically to the unique needs of organists.

Organ playing differs physically from piano playing in two basic areas:

1) Organists play on more than one keyboard. Those keyboards are on different levels, and one is often playing on more than one keyboard at the same time.
2) Organists use their feet to play the pedalboard, manipulate expression boxes, and push toe pistons. As a result, the feet are not firmly planted on the floor and thus cannot provide support or a feeling of being grounded. This has important

implications for matters of balance and for finding a proper sitting position. It also necessitates having a very clear understanding of how the feet, legs, and hip joints work.

Learning to play the organ musically and proficiently can require many years of careful practice and study. This study can be followed by a lifetime of playing, either professionally or for pleasure. Those years spent at the organ should be productive, enjoyable, rewarding, and pain free.

This book is about how we move our bodies to play the organ.

Thom Miles

Playing the piano

is

motion, emotion, and love.

CHAPTER 1: BASIC CONCEPTS

THE PROBLEM OF INJURY

Almost every pianist or piano teacher has experienced pain or knows someone who has experienced pain from playing the piano. Injuries are so common that some people believe pain is inevitable for pianists. A well-known teacher reportedly told an audience that "Pain is the price you pay for being a concert artist." But that is false. Playing the piano need not be painful. There are pianists who have played the most difficult literature throughout a lifetime with no problems.

Some people believe pain comes from being unlucky. Lucky pianists can play as much as they wish whereas unlucky pianists get injured. But that also is false. Musicians' injuries are not booby prizes in a lottery.

Pain in playing the piano can come from any of three causes. 1) It can come from a medical condition or illness, such as arthritis. 2) It can come from a trauma such as a sprain or fracture. Pain from either of these causes is appropriately treated by medical science. 3) Pain can come from inefficient use of the body—poor habits of movement. Almost all pain experienced by musicians falls in this third category. Pain caused by poor habits of movement is relieved by discovering and correcting those habits. If poor habits are not corrected, they can lead to injury, which in turn can cause permanent damage.

Playing any musical instrument requires repetitive motions. Piano playing is extremely repetitive. One handbook on stress injury considers any task requiring fifteen hundred repetitions per hour to be "highly repetitive." Fifteen hundred repetitions per hour may sound like a lot, but piano playing leaves it in the shade. The hourly rate of repetition for sixteenth notes at a metronome setting of a quarter note=120 is 28,800, a number that would doubtless cause apoplexy in a health inspector. In fact we *can* play sixteenth notes at 120, but we can't use just any motions to do it. A motion that involves even a small amount of tension can lead to injury when repeated thousands of times a day over a period of years. The elimination of musicians' injuries will come from education. When musicians and teachers know how to move safely and incorporate that knowledge into their playing and teaching, injuries will cease to be a problem.

Injury comes from playing with tension. "Tension" as used here means excessive muscular work—work in excess of what is needed to accomplish the task at hand. Tense ways of moving can be divided into general categories described in "The Four Causes of Injury" in Chapter 9. Tension can also come from social or cultural attitudes. For example, the prevailing beliefs about what counts as "good posture" produce tension. Pianists are as susceptible as anyone else to such cultural influences. But pianists are also at risk because some teaching methods condone or even inculcate tense ways of moving.

FINGER ORIENTATION

Some parts of traditional teaching of technique are perfectly sound. But other parts are false and dangerous. Unfortunately, what is harmful gets lumped together with what is sound and so is passed from one generation to the next. Thus, each generation has its share of injured pianists. To break out of this cycle we must separate what is safe from what is harmful, and reject what is harmful even when it is supported by authority and tradition.

Ironically, one of the most obvious facts about piano playing has also been an obstacle to understanding. The obvious fact is this: we play the piano with our fingers. The spectacle of a pianist's fingers at work has enthralled audiences throughout the history of the piano. An early example, the more telling since it comes from a novel, not a method book, is in Jane Austen's *Persuasion*, published in 1818. As Anne Eliot plays the piano, Mrs. Musgrove exclaims, "Well done, Miss Anne!…Lord bless me! how those little fingers of yours fly about!" (Book I, Ch. 6).

Since finger movements are obvious and other bodily movements used in piano playing are less obvious or seem to casual observers to be peripheral and not really necessary, people have tended to conclude that the fingers do most of the work of piano playing. This assumption also is reflected by Jane Austen. In *Pride and Prejudice* Elizabeth Bennet scores in a debate with Darcy by invoking the piano:

My fingers…do not move over this instrument in the masterly manner which I see so many women's do. They have not the same force or rapidity, and do not produce the same expression. But then I have always supposed it to be my own fault—because I would not take the trouble of practising. It is not that I do not believe *my* fingers as capable as any other woman's of superior execution (Vol. 2, Ch. 8).

If we play the piano with our fingers, it stands to reason that learning to play the piano is a matter of training our fingers. Consistent with this opinion, countless exercises have been devised in the name of strengthening the fingers, stretching the fingers, and developing independence of the fingers. C. L. Hanon, whose exercises are among the most widely used, speaks in his preface of training the fingers and claims that through his exercises "the fingers attain to an astonishing facility of execution." He does advocate "suppleness of the wrist," but that is the only part of the body besides the fingers that he so much as mentions.

Hanon is just one representative of a finger-oriented approach to piano playing that persisted throughout the nineteenth and twentieth centuries and seems unchallenged in the twenty-first. It is reflected in countless ways—a ragtime pianist with the nickname "Fingers," pieces with titles like "Dizzy Fingers," beginning piano books entitled *Fingerpower* or *Teaching Little Fingers to Play the Piano*. The examples are endless.

But we do not play the piano *only* by moving our fingers. Watch any pianist and you see numerous other movements. Arm movements. Torso movements. Leg movements. Playing the piano involves coordinated movement of many body parts. Overlooking these other movements is harmless in a casual conversation whose only purpose is to mention what is most obvious. But a teaching method based on finger movements isolated from supporting movements in the rest of the body is not harmless. It is dangerous.

Saying that we play the piano with our fingers is like saying that we run with our feet. The fingers move when we play the piano and they are the only parts of our upper body that touch the piano. Similarly, our feet move when we run and are the only parts that touch the ground. But a runner who tried to improve his running by keeping his legs motionless and doing foot exercises would be ridiculous. He is similar to a pianist who keeps his arms motionless and exercises his fingers, although what the pianist does has the sanction of tradition. We play the piano just as we run: by complex coordinated movements of our whole bodies.

THE MOVEMENT APPROACH

Numerous investigators have examined the physical movements of piano playing. Two important names in the early twentieth century are Tobias Matthay in England and Otto Ortmann in Germany. In the mid-twentieth century, a New York piano teacher named Dorothy Taubman made a huge contribution to the understanding of bodily coordination in playing the piano. Taubman observed that playing the piano is easy for some people, difficult for others. She saw that some pianists play for a lifetime with no problems whereas others are injured. She concluded that the pianists who play with ease and avoid injury must be doing something different from the others. She identified some of the subtle differences between the way the freest pianists moved and the way others moved. She recognized that certain ways of moving at the piano—those, for example, that involve co-contraction (which she called "dual muscular pulls"), chronic ulnar deviation

Organists too are often the unwitting victims of traditions passed down through generations of teachers. Some of these traditions, frequently found in method books, advocate moving only at the fingers while keeping the rest of the body perfectly still. It is understandable how this tradition gained popularity since the action of most organs is much lighter than the action of a typical piano. But finger orientation which excludes other movement can be just as harmful at the organ as it can at the piano.

(which she called "twisting"), or excessive force—are limiting and potentially injurious (these topics will be discussed in Chapter 9). Therefore, a safe technique will avoid those ways of moving. The value of Taubman's approach is shown by the many injured pianists who have been cured by adopting it and the many other pianists who, though never injured, have achieved new levels of skill.

Dorothy Taubman did not invent a new way to play the piano. She observed what was already done by pianists who played with fluency and ease. But unlike many other piano pedagogues she did not base her approach on the authority of those players— "so and so plays this way so you should, too"—but on the underlying anatomical facts. By taking into account the anatomy of the fingers, hands, and forearms and considering the ways in which movement can be easy or difficult, tense or free, she described ways to accomplish pianistic tasks using a better quality of movement.

The enormous difference that the quality of our movement makes in physical tasks, in sports, and in everyday life has gained recognition in recent decades. Many common aches, pains, and injuries that were formerly treated as medical problems or the inevitable consequences of age are now known to derive entirely or in part from a person's habits in using the body. That is to say, they have a *somatic* origin (from the Greek *soma*, meaning "body"). Physical problems with a somatic origin tend not to respond to ordinary treatments and therapies. Instead, they are improved or cured when the person learns a better quality of movement. Dorothy Taubman's results with both injured and non-injured pianists are an

example of what becomes possible when the physical task of piano playing is analyzed from the perspective of biomechanically efficient movement.

One of the pioneers in the field of movement reeducation was F. M. Alexander (1869-1955), who identified characteristic patterns of tension that interfere with breathing, speaking, and moving, sometimes causing severe impairment of those functions. He developed methods of teaching a better quality of movement and he trained others to teach his methods. The Alexander Technique is now taught by thousands of teachers throughout the world. Other important contributions have been made by Hans Seyle, Moshe Feldenkrais, Thomas Hanna, and Mabel Todd.

Musicians' injuries are almost always of somatic origin. They come from inefficient or stressful habits of movement. Change those habits and the problems disappear. This sounds easy but isn't always. Often, the only movements an injured pianist knows to use in specific instrumental tasks are the very movements that have led to injury. But that does not prove that there are no safe movements for these tasks. Pianists using other movements accomplish the same tasks without injury.

That seems obvious, but most pianists do not conclude that if there is pain there must be something wrong. Instead, believing that their technique is adequate, they pin the blame elsewhere—on overuse, perhaps, instead of misuse. They say, "I've been playing too much," not "I've been playing incorrectly." Instead of looking for appropriate help, they conclude, "I just overdid it and

I need to take it easy." One pianist told me that the problems for which she was wearing a brace on her wrist came from "too much Rachmaninoff." The fact is that pianists whose technique rests on a good quality of movement can play Rachmaninoff as much as they like.

✧ QUALITY OF MOVEMENT

Piano playing that is accomplished by high-quality movement, in which each part contributes its proper share with no tension, will be free, expressive, and secure. Playing that is accomplished by poor quality of movement, with tension, fatigue, and stiffness, will be insecure and unreliable.

It is best to think of quality of movement as a continuum, with high quality of movement at one extreme and poor quality at the other. Most actual movement falls somewhere in the middle, neither absolutely free nor completely tense. As the quality of movement improves, the playing becomes freer, more expressive, more secure, less likely to cause injury. As the quality of movement deteriorates, the playing becomes less secure, less expressive, more dangerous.

If one part of the body becomes fixed or stiff and ceases to contribute its share of the movement, we will probably still be able to play the piano. Other body parts will compensate. By working a little harder they can get the task accomplished. We can still play, but with a poor quality of movement.

Saying that someone plays with a poor quality of movement is not the same as saying that the *playing* is poor. Quality of movement and quality of playing are *connected,*

and improving the quality of movement will improve the playing and also overcome injury. But the two are not the same. Some people succeed in playing well, for a time, despite poor quality of movement.

That is, some people have a technique that includes inefficient, stressful movements. Nevertheless, with a powerful musical conception, by practicing diligently, forcing, and generally working very hard, they compensate for the inefficiencies and play well. Perhaps they even become virtuosos. But the outstanding playing may be obtained at a cost that the body cannot sustain indefinitely. There are people who play fabulously well—until they're injured and can't play at all.

This is a vital point, because people assume that anyone who plays beautifully must have an exemplary technique that can serve as a model for others. "Such and such a famous pianist did it this way" is taken to imply "It's OK to do it this way." But what if the famous pianist was injured? Not everyone knows that Glenn Gould, Sergei Rachmaninoff, Artur Schnabel, and many other famous pianists were injured.[1] Their injuries indicate that their techniques were flawed from a movement point of view. Obviously, we should acknowledge and emulate their artistic achievements, but it would be dangerous to model our technique uncritically on theirs.

---

[1] Rachmaninoff's injuries are described in his letters, particularly letters from the summer of 1923 in which he refers to the upcoming concert season as his "season of pain." Gould's injuries are described, in idiosyncratic terminology that makes diagnosis problematic, in his diaries, which have been studied by the neurophysiologist Frank R. Wilson. Wilson surmises that Gould's injury was dystonia. Schnabel refers in his memoirs to his "neuritis," which he calls his "occupational disease."

It is important at this point to offer a word of caution to organists (and harpsichordists) about relying on treatises, paintings, woodcuts, or other historic sources as a basis for hand position and/or movement at the keyboard. While these early sources often contain a wealth of important information useful for musical interpretation, it is dangerous to assume that accurate information about movement or hand position can be gleaned from such sources. It is likewise dangerous to rely on traditions passed down from studio to studio over a period of generations. For example, one person may have studied with another person who studied with a third person who said that J.S. Bach or Widor hardly moved at all while playing the organ.

In repetitive tasks it is vitally important to move well. Moving well is safe, moving badly is dangerous. Mere outward appearance does not always enable us to distinguish safe and dangerous movement. Two movements of the hand or fingers may look outwardly similar, and yet one may be free and easy, the other stiff and tense. The quality of one movement may be better than the quality of the other despite their similar appearance. This point is important because it is the quality of the movement, not its outward appearance—*how* we do it, not *what* we do—that makes the difference between free, expressive playing and limited, potentially injurious playing.

Playing the piano involves playing thousands of notes per hour and is appropriately regarded as a repetitive task. However, there is a vital sense in which piano playing is not repetitive, or not as repetitive as it appears. When I play the piano, the motion is not repetitive in the literal sense of repeating precisely the same motion over and over. I do not repeat the same note, played with the same motion of the same finger, over and over and over. I play different notes, at varying dynamic levels, using different fingers. This means that I am actually using *different* motions for each note. Even tiny variation in the movement can remove it from the category "repetitive." It's a different movement, using muscles differently, creating different forces in the connective tissue and using subtly different movement at the joints. Different composers require different movements, because they require different sounds. A safe player looks different playing Brahms from the way she looks playing Bach or Brubeck. An injured player usually looks just the same. Every piece of music consists of a series of notes different from any other piece of music (otherwise it wouldn't be a different piece), so every piece requires its own series of movements. It is appropriate to insist, as some teachers do, that the movement should be as complex as the music.

Complex, varied movement is indeed what we see in free players. But it is not usually what we see in injured players. Where free pianists make thousands of movements, injured pianists make hundreds. They use stereotyped movements instead of varied movements. If we see an injured pianist's movement speeded up on a video we can see how unnecessarily repetitive it is. Stereotyped movement makes piano playing more repetitive than it needs to be and is an important cause of injury.

Some widely accepted ways of teaching technique actually train a poor quality of movement, not a good one. This is true of the coin-on-the-back-of-the-hand (now thankfully out of fashion), also of the "finger independence" or "isolation" exercises in which one finger is moved while others are held motionless, and the exercises for stretching the fingers. Sometimes the problem comes from the notes of the exercise, those, for example, that demand spreading the fingers apart in attempted defiance of anatomy. More often the problem lies not in the notes of the exercise but in the instructions on how to practice. For example, the student may be told "keep your arm perfectly still and move only the finger" (that's what I was told). But that guarantees tense movement. Holding the arm still is accomplished by tensing it, and then, with the arm fixed and tense, the finger must work much harder. Such training brings about stereotyped movement. Someone who diligently follows those instructions will acquire a small repertoire of tense movements instead of a huge repertoire of free movements adaptable to any pianistic situation.

If a pianist has made poor-quality movements into a way of life and incorporated them into a technique, then telling that pianist (in the words of one book on piano technique) to "pace yourself to avoid any buildup of tension or fatigue" is fatuous. It is impossible advice to follow and it distracts attention from the real source of the problem, namely that the movements the pianist has learned are inherently dangerous.

Rather than focus just on specific movements, in the manner of so many exercise regimens, we need to be acutely aware of the quality of movement. Is the movement tense or free? Awkward or smooth? Easy or difficult? Many pianists are not aware of their bodies as they play, and therefore not aware of how they move their bodies. If you ask them, "How much of your body were you aware of as you played that passage? How much of your arm in addition to your fingers?" they may point to their forearm or their elbow as the boundary of their awareness.

Such limitation of awareness is actually dangerous. For example, many pianists complain of shoulder pain. Typically, they fix or set their collarbones and shoulder blades when they play, which involves tension. But they are not aware of the tension as they play, because they are not aware of their upper torso at all—until pain compels attention. If they learn to expand their awareness to include more of their bodies, that expanded awareness alone can produce improved quality of movement and better playing. So part of the answer to the question "How do we train a better quality of movement?" is that we do it by training attention and awareness. The full answer is more complex. Training the quality of movement involves attention and awareness combined with refinement of the kinesthetic sense and development of an accurate, adequate body map. I turn now to those essential concepts.

THE KINESTHETIC SENSE

I have just claimed that as we cultivate awareness, the quality of our movement improves. Why should that be? The answer lies in the feedback provided by our kinesthetic sense, a sense that many people are not even aware they have.

We ordinarily think of ourselves as having five senses: sight, hearing, taste, touch, and smell. That's what we were taught as children. But we actually have an additional sense, a sixth sense. The expression "sixth sense" usually refers to insight or intuition. But insight and intuition are not sensory modalities at all. I am talking rather of a genuine sensory mechanism different from the ones we colloquially recognize. That we have such a sense is clear from the following example. Suppose you and I each hold one hand above our head. I can see your hand but not my own. I cannot touch, see, smell, hear or taste the hand I am holding above my head, yet I know, by feeling, whether it is in the same position as yours. That is, we can know things about our bodies without deriving the information from any of the traditionally named senses. This information is sensory information in the strict sense: we have special nerve endings, mostly in our joints and connective tissue, that gather information about our position and our movement. The nerves that send this information to the brain are not the same as those that convey other sensory information—about sights, odors, sounds, tastes, and textures. These nerves convey information about *movement*. It is therefore appropriate to refer to this sensory modality as our "movement sense," or *kinesthesia,* or the *kinesthetic sense.*

Our kinesthetic sense informs us of the position and movement of our bodies. That is, it gathers and transmits information. But what we do with the information is not predetermined. We may use it or we may not. We may develop habits of attending to the information or habits of not attending. If our attention is elsewhere, information supplied by the kinesthetic sense goes unnoticed and unused. The situation is exactly similar to what happens with our other senses when we concentrate our attention elsewhere. If I am absorbed in reading a book I may be unaware of music in the background. Of course, the vibration of the air enters my ears and triggers a nervous signal that is sent to my brain and to that extent I "hear" the music. But if I do not attend to the sound, the music is not part of my awareness. If someone asks me later, "Did you like that music?" I may say, "What music? I didn't hear any music."

Similarly, if I play the piano and concentrate just on the action of my fingers, I may be completely unaware of tension or movement in my back and neck. The information is being sent to my brain through the sense receptors of my kinesthetic sense, but I am not aware of the information since I'm not attending to it. As a result, the information cannot function as *feedback,* to which I could respond by releasing my back and neck. My back and neck are tense and fixed, but I don't know it. My playing is less good than it could be, but I don't know that either. If I do hear shortcomings in my playing I won't identify the cause as upper body tension and I will probably try to improve my playing by continuing to concentrate on the action of my fingers. Thus, in my attempt to improve my playing I just make matters worse. By working my fingers harder I am attempting to compensate for stiffness and lack of appropriate movement elsewhere in my body. My practicing is a practicing of compensations—things that are necessary only because the quality of my movement is poor. Many pianists spend most of their time practicing compensations.

A word to organists. Amazingly, many of us are often aware of only the hands and feet and nothing in between. Imagine a snake with feeling and awareness in only its head and tail, or a cat that had no awareness of its front legs! Without an awareness of the pelvis and rockers, there can be no balance. Another problem can arise when playing a piece for manuals only. Some organists are aware of only the upper part of the body, ignoring the legs and feet and often the pelvis. When playing the piano, the feet are grounded on the floor. For an organist playing manuals only, however, becoming disembodied in the legs leads to a loss of awareness in the pelvic area, a loss of feeling grounded on the rockers, and an attempt to shift support of the upper body into the back and shoulders. Playing the organ comfortably and efficiently requires whole-body awareness, inclusive attention from head to toe and from fingertip to fingertip.

TRAINING ATTENTION

Pianists are sometimes urged to "concentrate on the music." This is not what I mean by attention. Concentration is not a solution—it is part of the problem. Concentration means directing attention to one thing and shutting out everything else. Concentrating on one thing, even something as important as the music, excludes the numerous other things that also affect our performance, such as the quality of our movement.

I urge that we banish "concentration" from our musical vocabulary and think instead of training attention. We need to attend to movement throughout our bodies as we play the piano. We need to be aware of our bodies as unified wholes. That is because *parts of the body that are not included in our awareness are likely to become fixed.* They will not contribute properly to the movement of the whole. When we expand our awareness to include the parts that have been fixed and stiff, they come alive. We can notice tension and release it. We respond to the information supplied by our kinesthetic sense and we recognize that one movement is free and easy, another stiff and difficult. We begin automatically to make the corrections that bring about a better quality of movement.

The appropriate mental state for musicians is one of inclusive attention. We need to develop a field of awareness that includes all the things that bear on our playing, not just our hands and arms but our backs and legs and entire bodies. Within this field of awareness we can focus as necessary on whatever requires attention at the moment. We play a passage and notice a hint of tension building in our neck, so we release it. The music requires us to play in the upper range of the keyboard and our body automatically moves there, giving a sense of balance and security. Gradually we become sensitive, discerning, responsive observers of ourselves.

In order to evaluate the quality of our movement we need to know what to look for. Attending to our movements without proper information may just serve to reinforce our current habits, since we are likely to call "good" whatever we are accustomed to. Thus, we may consider a movement acceptable because it is what we're used to, even though the movement really is potentially injurious. Another possibility is that we know that a certain way of moving doesn't feel good, but we don't know how to improve it or how to accomplish the pianistic task any other way. That is why telling students to play "naturally" or "do what feels natural" is so dangerous. Some teachers insist that they and their students cannot become injured because they play "naturally." All too often, they are wrong.

Good movement is indeed "natural" in two senses. First, it is natural in the sense that it is in harmony with the structure of the body. It is what we are "designed" for. Second, good movement is natural in the sense that it "comes naturally" when we are first learning to use our bodies. Most young children move efficiently and in balance. Alexander teachers often point to toddlers and preschool children as models of good use of the body.

But although good use is "natural" in the senses just given, it is not "natural" in the sense of feeling "normal" to someone whose habits are poor. People may stand badly, sit

badly, and move badly, yet the way they stand, sit, and move feels "natural" (i.e., normal) to them. To such a person, efficient movement will feel odd and unaccustomed (even if the person recognizes that it is better). Telling a student to do what feels right without demonstrating what actually *is* right usually amounts to reinforcing bad habits and is therefore poor teaching.

On the other hand, if we develop accurate knowledge of the structure of our bodies and the ways that structure allows for efficient movement, we can use the information to develop our kinesthetic sense. We can evaluate and improve the quality of our movement. This is the great insight of "Body Mapping." An accurate body map gives us the foundation for improved movement.

༄

THE BODY MAP

Suppose I stop at a red light and my ankle itches. Keeping my eyes on the light, I reach down and scratch the place that itches. Later, at a gas station, I reach under the seat and pull the lever to release the gas cap. Actions like these occur all the time. But they are remarkable. How do we know to put our hands in places we cannot see and perform specific actions? How do we know how far to lift our legs when climbing stairs in the dark?

Our ability to perform these actions shows that we have some practical knowledge of our body in movement. We evidently know something about our size, the weight and relative position of our parts, where the joints are, and how they move. That is to say, we have an internal representation of our body and its movements and we use this representation to coordinate our actions. This internal representation is our body map.

Our body map includes the structure, size, and function of our body and its parts. It is not something we are born with, nor does it remain fixed throughout our lives. It could not be fixed and still be useful. A boy's body map, representing a person four feet tall, would not work well when the boy has become a man six feet tall. It is ridiculous to imagine a tall man climbing a stepladder to reach the top of the refrigerator, as he did when he was five. But if his body map had not changed as he grew, that is what he would do. We generate our body maps from our experience and revise them through the course of our lives.

Like other experiential knowledge, our body map may be vague or detailed, accurate or inaccurate. More precisely: my body has a certain structure and it can move in specific ways. My representation of that structure—my body map—may accurately reflect the structure, or it may not. This is an important issue because our body map is a representation that governs our movement. That is, we move our bodies according to the way we think of them, not necessarily according to the way they actually are. This is true even if we have never consciously formulated our beliefs about our structure.

 We can put the point this way: our body has a particular anatomical structure. In our brain is a representation of that structure. But the representation, not the structure, determines how we try to move. If our body map is incorrect, we will try to move in a way inconsistent with the actual structure of our body. We will not succeed in changing our structure to fit our false beliefs. Instead, movement will be tense or awkward. Tension detracts from our piano playing. More than that, it is actually dangerous. That is, an inaccurate body map may lead us to move with tension that takes the form of one of the causes of injury described in Chapter 9 of this book.

Just as a poor body map generates poor quality of movement, an improved body map generates an improved quality of movement. How do we improve our body map? In the first place, we improve it by acquiring accurate anatomical information. This book aims to present the information that is important for pianists. Any information in this book that is new or surprising to you represents an opportunity to revise your body map, which will improve your quality of movement and the quality of your playing.

ॐ

THE BODY MAP VS. INTELLECTUAL KNOWLEDGE

Acquiring accurate anatomical information is not the same as developing an accurate body map. The body map is the self-representation that governs movement. A person may know about the structure of the body, but if that knowledge does not govern the person's movement, it is mere knowledge—not part of the person's body map. (Think of the anatomists and physicians who know lots of anatomy but move badly.) Conversely, someone can have an adequate and accurate body map without much conscious knowledge of anatomy. Some pianists move well intuitively, without deliberately having developed their body maps. Their body maps developed naturally and effortlessly, based on their experience of playing the piano.

The information presented in this book is essential for pianists, but it will make a difference to a person's playing only if it is incorporated into the person's body map. Acknowledging the information as true is not enough; the information must be profoundly integrated so that the new truth, not the old untruth, governs movement. Sometimes this can happen quickly, even overnight ("oh, *that's* how it works!"). Usually it is a gradual process involving a period of assimilation and conscious cultivation of new habits of moving. This requires consistency and perseverance and it brings a change in the way we perceive ourselves at the piano. Gradually, mere knowledge leads to an improved body map and the new movements become habits. As a valuable supplement to the information in this book, I encourage everyone to read the section entitled "Your Body Map and How to Change It" in Barbara Conable's *How to Learn the Alexander Technique.*

Throughout the book I urge readers to cultivate experience, not just absorb information. I offer "exercises" intended to help develop awareness and reinforce new habits. A person who merely reads and does not incorporate the information into the body map will learn some interesting facts but will not notice much improvement in piano playing. If that person is injured, the injury will persist.

FEELING EMBODIED

Many pianists are unaware of their torso, back, pelvis, or other body parts as they play. People who habitually ignore their bodies, or parts of their bodies, as they go about their activities may develop what I shall call "disembodiment." They are out of touch with their own bodies. A disembodied person may have trouble bringing the body, or parts of the body, into awareness; may use excessive force because of inability to feel just how much work is needed; may be at a loss when asked to describe sensations in the arm or hand. Often such people are more accident-prone than others. Sometimes they become aware of the body only when awareness is forced by pain.

Disembodiment is a disaster for pianists. Pianists need to be aware of their bodies. This awareness needs to be vivid, inclusive, and specific to the individual, a sense of *my* body. "My body has a particular structure and way of moving; I move this body, structured this way, to play the piano." The immediate, detailed awareness of the body is what I am calling "feeling embodied" or "being embodied."

Being embodied is crucial for free, non-injurious playing. As we know, injury and limitation come from stressful moving. Stressful moving may result from one or both of two factors: 1) lack of awareness of the body and 2) mismapping the structure and movement of the body. This book presents the information needed to correct mismapping. We have pointed out before that mere information is powerless until, through the activity of Body Mapping, it becomes part of the person's body map. We can now make this last point differently: the information must contribute to the sense of embodiment. In other words, having learned the facts about my body's structure and movement, I must make those facts the basis of my sense of embodiment. Then my sitting, breathing, playing of scales and octaves will all be organized in a balanced, efficient way. Achieving this may take time, and for people who have a habit of disembodiment it will not happen automatically. It must be chosen and cultivated. Attention is the key.

Attend to tactile sensations of all kinds—itchiness, warmth, cold. Add other tactile experience such as your clothes on your body, your hands touching your body or each other. Then attend to kinesthetic experience, your movement, position, and size. Attend to the delivery of weight to the chair seat, the floor, the back of the chair. Locate yourself throughout your body, in your legs, hands, lungs, and everywhere.

Here is an example illustrating the value of developing the feeling of embodiment. Often in teaching we have occasion to ask a pianist, "How much of your body were you aware of as you played that passage?" If the pianist looks puzzled, we may elaborate, "I suppose you were aware of your fingers and your hands. Were you also aware of your wrists? Your forearm? Your upper arm? Your torso? How much of your body was included in your awareness?" Often, the pianist claims awareness of nothing further back than the elbow. Our next step is to encourage the pianist to become aware of—that is, to attend to—the whole arm (and ultimately, the whole body). We may

have the pianist move the arms around a bit, paying attention to all four major joints, to stimulate awareness, and then play the passage again. The passage invariably sounds better than before.

I have already pointed out the dangers and limitations of the "finger-oriented" approach to playing the piano. I claimed that we need to move away from "I move my fingers to depress the keys" to "I move my body to play the piano." The concept of embodiment permits us to go one step further, to "I move my embodied self to make music."

~

KINESTHETIC AND MUSICAL IMAGINATION

The final assertion in the last paragraph—that we move our embodied selves to make music—is profoundly important. It means that when our awareness of our bodies in movement is based on refined kinesthesia and a good body map, our conception of the music—the sound—will fuse with our conception of the movement that produces the music. Putting the point slightly differently: when we conceive a musical result, that conception will instantly translate into a kinesthetic awareness of the movement that brings about the result. Our musical conception will be realized, in sound, through movement. Refining and deepening our musical ideas will elicit ever more refined and subtle movement. Practicing will become a matter of conceiving a sound, then discovering and practicing the movements that produce the sound. This uniting of musical and kinesthetic imagination depends on developing kinesthesia, a sense of embodiment, and a good body map, but thinking in these terms from the outset will help you develop those things. As you progress along this path, the musical imagination and the kinesthetic imagination can feed on each other, assisting each other to higher and higher levels.

BRAINWORK

Some people think of playing the piano as mainly a physical skill. Others insist that it must come from the heart and the emotions. In fact, it is both, and more besides. Playing the piano is one of the most complex of human activities. Our brains have several distinct functional areas. There is the cognitive function, which is the process of knowing and remembering; the sensory function, which governs sensation including kinesthesia; the motor function, which controls movement; and the emotional function, which relates to feelings. Some activities may use just one of these functions, but all of them are combined in piano playing. The brain must coordinate them, bringing them together, simultaneously, when we play. Playing the piano is brainwork, and pianists need to be constantly aware of the different functional areas of the brain they call on in their playing. Not just in a general way, but in specific ways, all the time. If I don't do that, I'll just be playing notes—that is, I'll be treating piano playing as a merely physical skill, which would be to trivialize it. I must learn to relate the emotional content of the music, at every moment, to my physical kinesthetic sensations and the movements of my body that produce music from the piano. I must map emotion as sensation and movement.

HOW TO USE THIS BOOK

This book is intended to present information and to be used as an aid in the activity of Body Mapping. Pianists should read and understand the information. Then they should actively map the information in their own bodies as needed.

As you read, locate the bones and joints in your own body. Touch them, palpate them, massage them, move them. Develop your kinesthetic sense and learn to be directly aware of many joints and structures that most people do not pay much attention to— the head on the spine, the shoulder joints, the lumbar spine, the hip joints. Continue doing this until the feeling of yourself as a body with *this* structure, balanced *this* way, and with *these* possibilities of movement, is completely assimilated.

Keep the book open on the piano to a different page each day. Throughout that day's practice, refer back to it over and over to refine your awareness of the movements and structures shown. Make photocopies of the illustrations and post them on your bathroom mirror, your front door, your refrigerator—places where you'll see them constantly. Whenever you see the pictures consult your kinesthetic sense and ask, "Am I aware of that structure in its proper free relation to the rest of me?" (and be sure the question you ask yourself is "Am I aware of?" not just "Do I know about?").

A pitfall that is extremely easy to fall into, especially for pianists who are not injured (so pain does not sound an alarm), is that they sit down, think briefly about sitting in balance or releasing their shoulders, and proceed to practice for an hour with no further attention to the body. New habits have been reinforced for 30 seconds, old habits for 59 minutes 30 seconds. An injured pianist who practices this way will not recover, and a non-injured pianist will not experience the transformation in playing that this information enables.

A pianist cultivating a better way of moving must make that the first priority of each practice session. For a while it must take priority over learning new repertoire, preparing for a performance, etc. The goal is that every note be the product of a coherent, efficient movement based on an accurate, adequate body map and that the pianist be aware of it as such. For injured pianists the process may be slow at first. An injured pianist may need to begin with practice sessions of only five minutes.

Interrupt your practice sessions frequently, perhaps using a mechanical timing device, to refresh your awareness of the balance and structure of those parts of your body that you formerly mismapped and are now remapping. You must do this regularly and make this sort of practicing into a consistent habit to experience the astonishing power of the information in this book.

Throughout the book I include suggestions for developing body awareness and improving quality of movement. These suggestions for active participation are usually presented in italics. The movements and thought experiments are intended to encourage the self-exploration that leads to greater awareness and an improved body map.

✧

LESSONS

Any motivated pianist can make progress using this book. Many musicians have transformed their playing unaided by anything but learning the truth about their structures and actively imitating healthy movement. However, almost all pianists, especially injured pianists, will do well if possible to have at least a few lessons with someone trained in this material. A teacher can accelerate the process, point out things that the pianist may not be aware of, guide the pianist to solutions and show how to find solutions to future problems. This personal guidance can be very helpful and encouraging. For injured pianists, who are often discouraged or depressed, the support of a sympathetic, informed teacher is invaluable.

CHAPTER 2: MAPPING THE STRUCTURE

The body map is the internal representation in the brain that governs movement. *Body Mapping* (designated in this book with capital letters) is not the same thing. Body Mapping is an *activity* in which, through the training of attention and the refinement of kinesthesia, information ceases to be "external" and becomes "internal"—part of the representation in the brain governing movement. The distinction between the body map and Body Mapping is reflected in the titles of this and subsequent chapters. The title of this chapter is not "Structure" but "Mapping the Structure," the next chapter is not "Places of Balance" but "Mapping the Places of Balance." The purpose of the titles is to remind readers to approach the information actively. This is a workbook, not a textbook.

ॐ

SUPPORTING AND DELIVERING WEIGHT

When we stand or sit upright we are supported by the bony structure of our bodies. In holding us upright the structural parts of the body play a dual role: they *support* the parts above them, from which they receive weight, and they *deliver* weight to the parts (or the ground) below them. Since supporting and delivering weight is what the structure is designed for, uprightness is not something we need to bring about consciously. It is not something we *do*, it happens because of the way we are built. The weight-bearing and weight-delivering capacity of the bony structure is what makes mechanical advantage possible.

It is useful to regard both functions—delivering weight and supporting weight—as active or dynamic functions. The head, for example, when in balance, delivers weight precisely and evenly to the top vertebra of the spine, which is designed to receive it. If the head is off balance, it will deliver weight unevenly, to the wrong place, or in the wrong direction, obliging various muscles to work in compensation. If imbalance becomes chronic, the muscular compensation becomes chronic also, restricting freedom of movement and, perhaps, creating other serious problems.

The supporting of weight is dynamic also. Physics tells us that the weight of an object (such as the skull) represents a force toward the center of the earth. To prevent the object falling, the force must be counteracted by an equal and opposite force. Therefore, the skull exerts a downward force that is exactly matched by the upward force coming from the spine. The upward force is something we can learn to feel. All too often, habits of chronic muscular tension make us unaware of the way our bony structure supports us. When we learn to sit and stand in balance, we can release some of that muscular effort. We can attend to and experience the support supplied from the ground and up through our bony structure as a dynamic upward force, a sort of "buoyancy." Cultivating this kind of balance makes movement easier and improves piano playing. A different way of putting the point is this: when we learn to rely on the bony structure and the automatic postural adjustments to hold us up (instead of thinking we need to use muscular work), tension can be released and we are free to approach piano playing from a position of mechanical advantage.

This chapter describes the principal weight-bearing and weight-delivering structures in the body. The next chapter, "Mapping the Places of Balance," examines the interrelation of those structures in balance and movement. The emphasis in this chapter is on *structures* and in the next chapter on *joints*.

৵

THE SKULL

The skull is massive and roughly spherical. It sits, balanced, on the top of the spine. Its weight is delivered to the structures below it. Since it is at the top of the body it does not support the weight of any other body part. The ear marks the approximate center, front to back, of the skull. With your thumb at your ear you can rotate your arm to move your index finger, like a compass tracing a circle with your thumb as the center, to verify that the ear is the center, front to back, of the skull.

The jaw is not part of the skull. It attaches to the skull at a joint in front of the ears (the temporo-mandibular joint or "TMJ"). The lower teeth attach to the jaw, which should move freely without disturbing the balance of the skull. The upper teeth do not attach to a second jaw, they attach to the base of the skull itself. Notice how easy it is to chew using the movement of the single jaw and how much tension is created if you imagine yourself with two moving jaws opening and closing like a trap.

Two common mapping errors are, first, thinking that the skull is supported somewhere toward the back instead of in the middle, and second, thinking that the head includes the jaw and the neck begins at the bottom of the jaw. A person who makes this second error develops a "head-neck unit" which hampers playing.

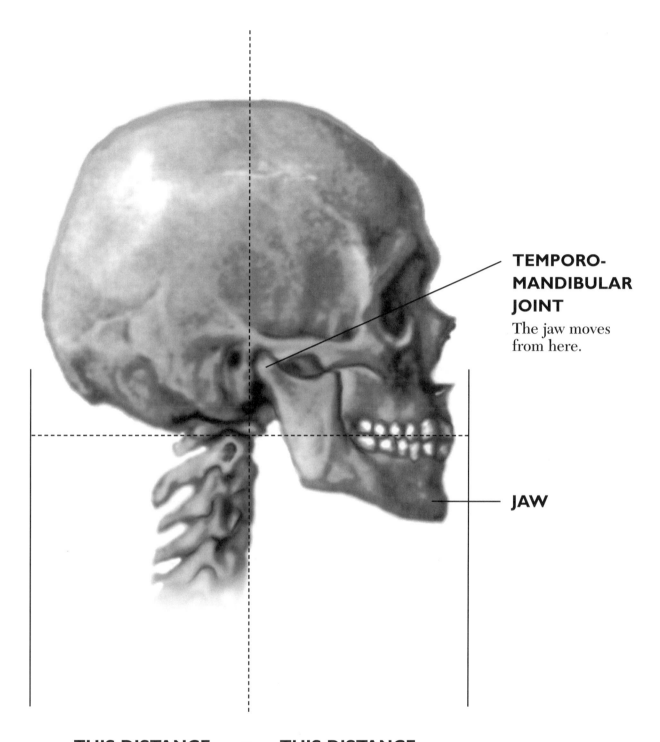

**TEMPORO-
MANDIBULAR
JOINT**
The jaw moves
from here.

JAW

THIS DISTANCE   =   THIS DISTANCE

The head balances at its center on the spine.
The upper teeth, not the jaw, are the reference
point for level balance of the skull.

BACK

FRONT

THE SPINE

The weight-bearing spine consists of twenty-four vertebrae. It is divided into three regions: the *cervical* (neck) region with seven vertebrae, the *thoracic* (chest) region with twelve vertebrae, and the *lumbar* (lower back) region with five vertebrae. Seen from the side, the spine has several curves. It curves slightly inward (forward) in the neck region, outward in the thoracic region, inward again in the lumbar region. The curves permit the spine to absorb impact.

The weight-bearing spine delivers weight to the top of the *sacrum,* a wedge-shaped piece of bone attached to the pelvis. The sacrum is generally considered to consist of five vertebrae fused together, which makes it part of the spine. But in its function the sacrum is part of the pelvis. It does not participate in spinal movement. It attaches to the pelvis where it receives weight from the weight-bearing spine and delivers the weight outward to the rest of the pelvic arch.

There are four vestigial vertebrae below the sacrum, the coccygeal vertebrae, which constitute our "tailbone." They provide attachments for muscles and ligaments. They do not bear weight. That is, they *should* not bear weight. Pianists who map their tailbones as bearing weight rock their pelvises backward. This drives the tailbone into the bench, producing inflammation and even the eventual breaking apart of the tailbone.

The front part of each vertebra is a cylindrical piece of bone, the *body* of the vertebra. Taken together, the bodies of the separate vertebrae form a curvy column with each

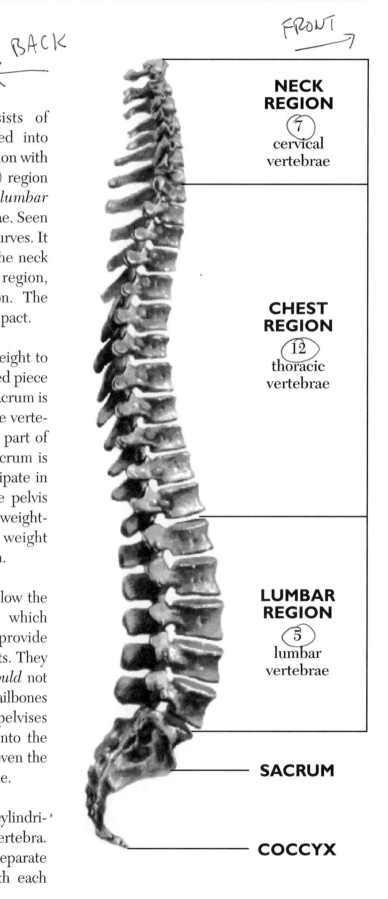

NECK REGION ⑦ cervical vertebrae

CHEST REGION ⑫ thoracic vertebrae

LUMBAR REGION ⑤ lumbar vertebrae

SACRUM

COCCYX

piece slightly bigger than the one above it. The vertebral bodies are separated by fibrous cushions or *discs.* The discs are elastic; they absorb shocks and allow for bending and twisting of the spine. The bodies of the vertebrae and the discs between them make up the weight-bearing part of the spine—our "core support."

The back part of each vertebra is a complicated structure consisting mostly of three protrusions of bone called *processes.* The processes serve to anchor muscles, and they include *facets,* which are the places where ribs attach or places where one vertebra is in contact with the adjacent vertebra. The facets prevent too great a range of motion. There is a hole in each vertebra called the *foramen.* The foramina of the vertebrae line up to form a tunnel through which the spinal cord runs. Between each pair of vertebrae a pair of nerves branches off the spinal cord to supply different parts of the body.

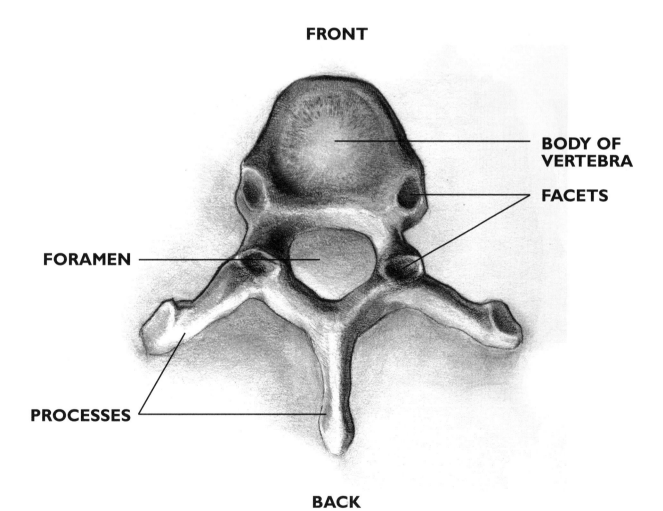

FRONT

BODY OF VERTEBRA

FACETS

FORAMEN

PROCESSES

BACK

Single vertebra seen from above.

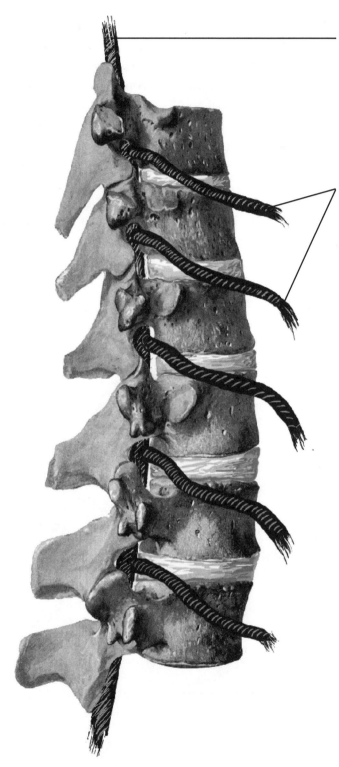

SPINAL CORD

Sends information
to and from the
brain.

NERVES

Send information to
and from
different parts
of the body.

Delivering weight
through the core
support keeps
pressure off the
nerves.

NERVE-HOUSING | WEIGHT-BEARING

The front and back portions of the spine look different from each other, because they perform different tasks. The front part supports and delivers weight. The back part houses nerves and anchors ribs. It is vital to grasp that the weight-bearing part of the spine is the *front* part of the spine. It is close to the center of the body. When we look at a person's back, the lumps we see and call the "backbone" are the tips of the processes.

They are not the weight-bearing part of the spine. People who think those lumps bear weight suffer back pain and tension. We can learn to be aware of support up through the center of us from the weight-bearing spine—our core support. The core support is *inside* our ribs. Being aware of the core support permits us to release back, chest, and arm muscles.

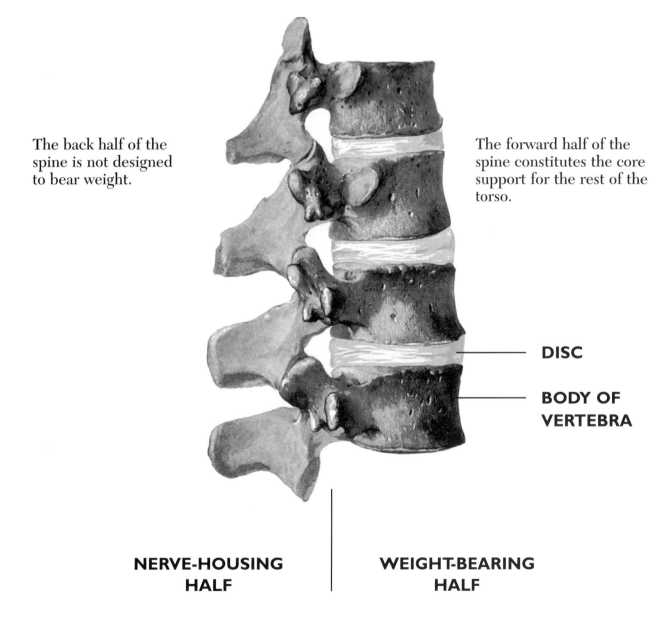

The back half of the spine is not designed to bear weight.

The forward half of the spine constitutes the core support for the rest of the torso.

DISC

BODY OF VERTEBRA

NERVE-HOUSING HALF

WEIGHT-BEARING HALF

Many people map their spines close to the surface of their backs. But as the above discussion makes clear, the weight-bearing part of the spine is not near the skin surface but deep inside the body, at the core. The distinction between *spine* and *back* is vital. In the lumbar region, the spine is not at the back but dead center in the body. People who imagine that the support from the spine is along the surface of the back instead of up through the middle of the body develop a "back-oriented" way of standing and sitting. They may throw the weight backward toward the tailbone, even though the tailbone is not designed to bear weight. Back orientation is extremely common among pianists, and extremely destructive.

Back orientation is almost epidemic among organists! Because the feet of an organist are not firmly planted on the floor, many organists feel unbalanced and compensate by distorting the natural shape of the spine into a large letter **C**, *and sitting, or attempting to sit, on the tailbone. The results are often disastrous as the legs and arm structure are robbed of their freedom to move freely and fluently. This will be discussed in more detail in the chapter "Mapping the Places of Balance."*

SPINAL MOVEMENT

The elasticity of the discs permits small movements of the vertebrae. These small movements, added up along the length of the spine, permit the spine to bend, twist, and spiral, with each disc absorbing some of the movement. Movement should not be concentrated more in one region of the spine than another; instead it should be distributed along the entire structure. Many pianists sit with the pelvis fixed. When they adjust to play in different areas on the piano, they move from the waist, as if the waist were a joint. This habit makes playing more difficult, and it can hurt. Another destructive habit is the head-neck unit, that is, the AO joint, where the head meets the spine, seems to be frozen and the head and neck move as a unit from the base of the neck. This is due to mismapping. It ruins spinal flexibility, compromises collarbone and shoulder blade movement, and hampers development of an inner sense of support for the arms in playing.

The elasticity of the discs permits the vertebrae to move farther apart and then come closer together again, resulting in a measurable and perceivable lengthening and gathering of the spine. (A teacher can see it; a student can feel it or, with cultivation of the kinesthetic sense, learn to feel it.) If the lengthening and gathering of the spine is not inhibited by tension, it occurs thousands of times a day, coordinating our breathing, our running, our walking, our bending and reaching, and our more complex activities like playing the piano.

Spinal lengthening and gathering is absolutely vital for pianists. That is because we can experience real support for the arms only if lengthening and gathering is occurring. Without it, pianists' arms feel heavy and "held up." With it, arms feel buoyed up. When the spine's lengthening and gathering is supporting them, the arms never feel isolated from the rest of the body. Rather, they are always felt to be in relationship to the spine, the bench, the floor, the whole body. If you feel that your arms are freely floating, not heavy or constrained in any way, not resting on anything, and you feel that the whole of you is the source of the sound, then you are very likely lengthening and gathering naturally already.

This lengthening and gathering is natural and intrinsic. It's just the way your body works when it isn't tensed. You naturally become greater in length as you, for instance, reach for a cup off a high shelf, and you naturally settle a bit in your spine as you put the cup on the counter, just as a cat gathers a bit to prepare to spring and lengthens a bit in the springing. "Lengthen" in this context means "to become greater in length," not "to make greater in length." If you try to *make* yourself greater in length in playing, you'll just end up confused and strained. If you *allow* yourself to become greater in length, you will feel buoyed up. How will you know when to lengthen and when to gather? The music will tell you. (If that sounds obscure, think of it this way: when you have a conception of the sound you want, your body, if you are fully embodied without tension, will automatically respond to execute the conception.)

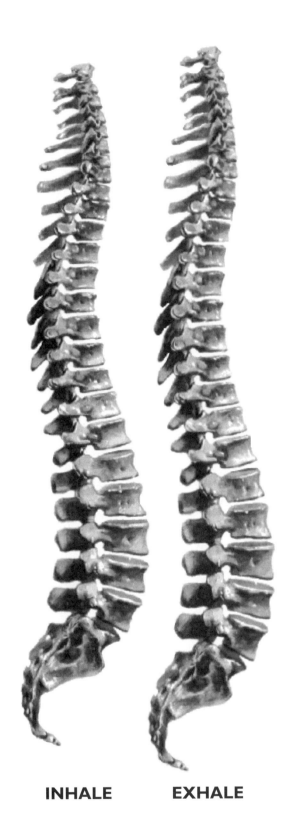

INHALE   **EXHALE**

When we are at rest, spinal lengthening and gathering is coordinated with breathing.

Pianists have more choice about when to lengthen and gather than other musicians. Singers must gather on inhalation and lengthen on exhalation. String players almost always gather on the upbow and lengthen on the downbow. Pianists have choices. They can lengthen or gather in response to the expressive choices they make about the music.

In well-coordinated movement, the head leads and the spine follows, so that individual vertebrae are moving sequentially. Watching a snake, which is nothing but head and spine, is illustrative. The snake leads with its head and the entire rest of the spine follows the head. Snakes and pianists are vertebrates. If the snake had limbs, its limbs would be coordinated by the spine. Pianists do have limbs, which are coordinated by the spine as the snake's would be.

The principles of efficient movement of the spine can be summed up as "The Laws of the Spine:"

1. The head leads.
2. The vertebrae follow in sequence.
3. Movement is distributed over the entire spine.
4. The spine must be free to lengthen and gather.

Pianists moving side to side and forward and back to play in different parts of the keyboard will find their movement effortless and enabling of the arms if they move in accordance with the Laws of the Spine. Pianists should recognize that the spine extends from the base of the head all the way down to the pelvis, and cultivate a sense of one whole, segmented spine which moves along its entire length. Movement should not be confined to any one part, nor should any part be held fixed.

Saying that the head leads is partly a description of what happens, partly a description of what we do: I lead, with my head, a motion that in the end includes my entire spine. It is not a thrusting of the head; the feeling is more like the head floating in the appropriate direction. If I do not lead with my head, then I will initiate somewhere else, with my chest, perhaps, and movement will not be as well organized. Spinal movement that is properly led by the head feels smaller, easier, and more secure and sequential than movement initiated some other way.

Some pianists fear that leading with the head to play at the extremes of the keyboard will leave the body unbalanced. There are two responses to this. One is to encourage the pianist to experiment and discover that when the head leads there is, in fact, no sense of being off balance. A second response is the reminder that the body includes the legs, and support from the legs is vital for creating a sense of balanced ease in movement. Leading with some part other than the head (the chest, for example) generally isolates the torso from the legs and the result is indeed a feeling of being off balance. When movement is led by the head, the legs contribute support and there is no sense of being off balance.

❧
THE PELVIS

The pelvis receives the weight of the upper body. The weight-bearing part of the pelvis is an arch with the sacrum as its keystone. Geometrically, an arch is a very efficient structure for bearing and delivering weight and we shall encounter it in other parts of the body. The sacrum receives weight from the lumbar spine and delivers weight through the arch of the pelvis to the legs when we are standing, or to the sitting bones (or "rockers") when we are sitting. If you examine a model of the pelvis you will discover that the weight-bearing and weight-delivering parts of the pelvis, the parts that coincide with the arch structure, are much thicker than the parts such as the iliac crest that do not bear weight. Weight is delivered to the legs through the hip joints, which are low on the sides of the pelvis. The joints are lower than many people think—about as low as the bottom of your briefs (if you wear briefs). When we sit, the legs bend at the hip joints and weight is delivered through the sit bones to the bench. (A detailed discussion of sitting is in Chapter 3.)

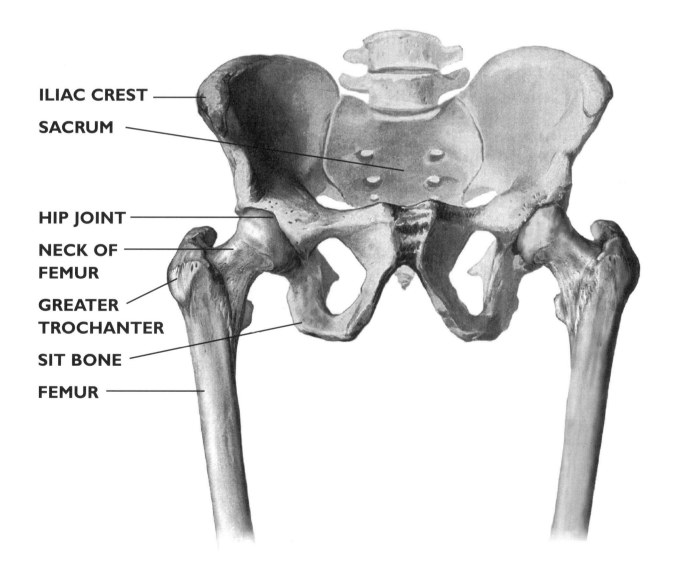

ILIAC CREST

SACRUM

HIP JOINT

NECK OF FEMUR

GREATER TROCHANTER

SIT BONE

FEMUR

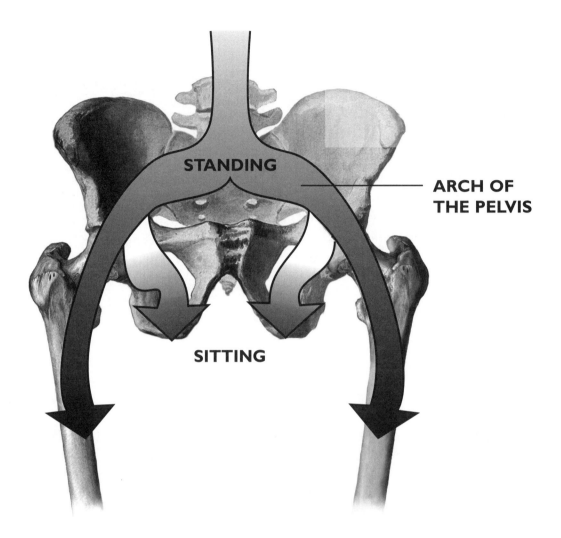

STANDING

ARCH OF
THE PELVIS

SITTING

Weight of the torso is delivered outward through
the hip joints to the thighbones when standing,
and downward to the sit bones when sitting.

❧

Organists take note. A clear understanding of the pelvis and sit bones is crucial for playing the organ. In most cases we do not have the luxury of using our legs for balance and support as we play. Instead, we are using our legs and feet to play the pedalboard, and to manipulate expression boxes and toe pistons. (A further discussion of sitting at the organ is in Chapter 3.)

❧
THE UPPER LEG

Our upper leg bone, the femur, takes the weight of the torso at the hip joint and delivers it to the lower leg at the knee joint. The upper end of the femur is made up of a *head* (the "ball" that fits the "socket" of the hip joint) and a *neck* that connects the head to the shaft of the femur. The head and neck angle sharply out to the side from the pelvis, making the top of the shaft of the femur (the *greater trochanter*) project further out to the side of the body than any part of the pelvis. The shaft of the femur, seen from the front, is not vertical when we stand (unless we stand with our legs spread apart). From the greater trochanter, it slants back toward the center axis of the body. Thus, a person's *leg* may appear vertical from the front, but the *bone* inside the thigh is slightly diagonal. That way, the knee joint, where the lower end of the femur connects with the shinbone, can be aligned directly below the hip joint. This arrangement—the neck of the femur extending to the side and the shaft slanting back toward the center—enhances the mobility of the hip joint and the stability of the body in standing.

❧
THE LOWER LEG

The lower leg has two bones, fixed parallel to each other. The *tibia* or "shinbone" is the large bone in front and the *fibula* is the small bone in back. You can feel the shinbone along its entire length just under the skin of the front of the lower leg. The shinbone is the weight-bearing bone. (The fibula cannot bear weight since its upper end does not even connect with the weight-delivering

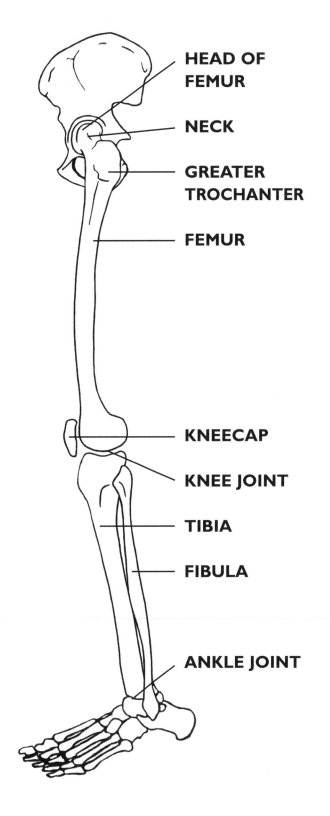

HEAD OF FEMUR

NECK

GREATER TROCHANTER

FEMUR

KNEECAP

KNEE JOINT

TIBIA

FIBULA

ANKLE JOINT

bone of the upper leg, the thighbone.) The shinbone receives the weight of the upper body from the thighbone at the knee joint and delivers it through the ankle joint to the foot.

Note that the knee *joint,* through which the shinbone receives weight from the thighbone, does not coincide with the knee*cap.* The knee joint is behind and slightly below the kneecap. The knee joint transmits weight; the kneecap does not bear weight.

THE FOOT

The foot receives the weight of the body from the femur at the ankle joint. The weight-bearing part of the foot is an arch. One end of the arch is the back of the heel bone, the other end is the ball of the foot (the toes are not part of the arch). The ankle joint is between the back of the heel and the ball of the foot, on the arch, at the front end of the heel bone. The arch distributes the

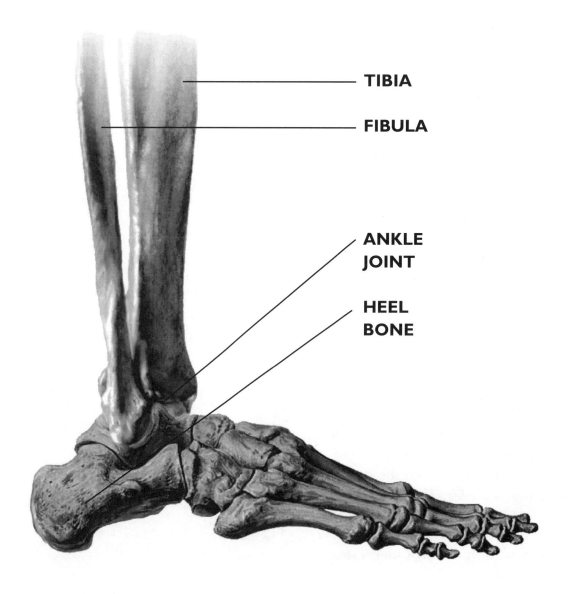

TIBIA

FIBULA

ANKLE JOINT

HEEL BONE

weight of the body forward and back: forward to the ball of the foot and backward to the heel. The ball of the foot has two weight-bearing areas, one behind the big toe and one behind the little toe (they are connected by a second, transverse arch). There are thus three weight-bearing areas in the foot: two in the ball of the foot and one at the heel. None of these receives the entire weight of the body when we stand. We can think of the foot as a three-legged platform or tripod (a very stable structure), and we stand on the middle of it, not on one of the edges.

It should be noted by organists that these three weight-bearing areas of the foot are precisely the three areas used for playing the pedals. A further discussion of pedal playing will follow in the chapter called "Additional Concerns of Organists."

CHAPTER 3: MAPPING THE PLACES OF BALANCE

❧

POSTURE VS. BALANCE

Conventional wisdom has it that we should "sit up straight" at the piano, we should not "slump" and we should not be "tense" or "rigid." Instead, we should be "relaxed," "balanced," "poised." But what do people mean by these recommendations? What must we do to "sit up straight"? The question is of vital importance because the answers most people take for granted are wrong and harmful. Our society is the victim of a host of misconceptions about posture. I shall call them Posture Myths. "Chest out, shoulders back, suck in your gut, flatten your butt…" These military-sounding admonitions pop into people's minds when they think of "good posture." They certainly are "posture" in one sense offered by my dictionary: "an affected or unnatural attitude, or a contortion of the body." But they are not good. They are not the source of free, easy movement but of tension, back pain, and misery. The Posture Myths—some people call them a "cultural virus"—should not only be discarded, they should be vigorously opposed. But what do we put in their place?

Many people expect standing or sitting to require continual work. For people who believe the Posture Myths, standing or sitting upright will indeed be an effort, for they must constantly hold muscles tense as they attempt to maintain the prescribed posture.

If standing and sitting are uncomfortable, the same people may imagine that muscles are weak and in need of strengthening, or that they have bad backs. But often there is nothing wrong except the way of sitting and standing. The solution does not lie in strengthening. It lies in developing an accurate body map and replacing "posture" with balance.

For a moment, imagine a structure that is not a human body. It is a construction made from an erector set. Imagine it to be about as tall as a person, with beams or "arms" moved by pulleys and strings. In order to stand, the structure must be in reasonable equilibrium. A vertical line drawn through its center of gravity must reach the floor within the space outlined by whatever supports it has—otherwise it will be out of balance and either fall or require outside support. But if it is in equilibrium, then nothing *else* is required to hold it up. That is: the pieces of the erector set, attached end to end, hold it up. They *are* the structure but they also *support* the structure.

The strings that activate the moveable parts of the structure do not hold the structure up. They just apply force at places on the beams, causing them to move. Notice further that if the strings are held continuously tight, the parts they move will be less mobile. The full range of motion of the parts will be restricted if the strings are not allowed to release. Furthermore, if the strings are held continuously tense, they will tend to pull parts of the structure together. That is, the structure will be subjected to forces pulling it down and in on itself. Depending on the structure's design, continual tension on the strings might cause it actually to change shape. Or it might retain its shape despite the tension, with reduced mobility.

Our bodies are analogous to the erector set construction. When we stand or sit upright in balance, our skeleton is largely self-supporting. The bones and connective tissue support our weight and conduct it to the ground (or the piano bench) with little need for muscular effort. We are poised, free to move in many ways, and the movement feels easy and effortless. Our postural reflexes automatically and effortlessly supply the adjustments needed to maintain balance. When we move, our muscles, just like the strings in the erector set, apply force at appropriate points, causing movement.

But if we fall into habits of imbalance, we must constantly use muscular tension to counteract the imbalance. When that happens, movement becomes less efficient because muscles that should be available for movement are being used for support. The chronic muscular tension that results from habits of imbalance restricts our movement and over time may distort our shape. Such distortions are very common.

⁓

DOWNWARD PULL

The suggestion that habits of imbalance may eventually distort our shape may seem farfetched. It will seem less farfetched if we consider that the head is quite a heavy object—about ten pounds—poised on top of the spine like a pumpkin on a broomstick. There are obvious advantages to having our heads at the top of our bodies. It is an eminently convenient arrangement, provided the head sits balanced directly above the structures that support it and receive its weight. Unfortunately, for many people, the head is not poised directly above the supporting structures. Instead, the neck habitually appears to be collapsed forward which puts the head in front of the center of gravity of the body. That might not matter if the head were tiny like the head of a brontosaurus, insignificant in relation to the rest of the creature. But the human head is heavy. If it is carried forward of balance, compensations must be made elsewhere in order for the person to remain upright.

Typical compensations are, first, to tense the muscles in the neck so the head can be horizontal and the eyes can look forward instead of downward. This brings the head level but still leaves the neck thrust forward; thus, the head remains off balance in relation to the rest of the body. To counterbalance the head and keep the body from falling over, the compensation is that the thorax gets pushed backward. That creates pressure in the lumbar spine, so the hips are thrust forward to relieve the pressure. When the hips move forward, the knees lock to retain stability. Thus, the head's going out of balance triggers a chain reaction of compensations throughout the body. These compensations mean that some muscles are chronically stretched, others chronically shortened. Over time, connective tissue—tendons, ligaments, and fascia—adapts to the compensations.[1]

[1] The pattern of compensations described in these paragraphs is common, but it is not the only pattern. Downward pull can take various forms.

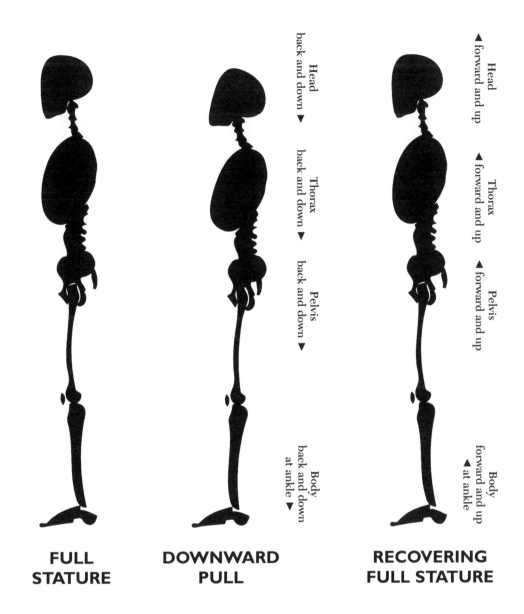

FULL STATURE

DOWNWARD PULL

RECOVERING FULL STATURE

All the compensations described above involve muscular tension, and all of them have a tendency to pull the body in on itself, making it shorter. This is what Alexander called "downward pull." It is common, even prevalent, in Western countries. Downward pull is implicated in many of the ailments—lower back pain, tension headaches, knee problems, and so on—that afflict people in our culture. It is dangerous for pianists also. That is because the compensations for imbalance in the upper body—tensing the neck, thrusting the chest backward, gripping in the lower back—all involve tensing muscles which, besides moving the neck, chest, etc., also control our arms. This means that if a pianist is out of balance, the muscular work of compensating for the imbalance inhibits the free movement of the arms.

The tension that results in downward pull is not usually perceived as tension. A person who exhibits the patterns of tension described above is unlikely to say, "I am tense;" the tension, after all, is chronic, and therefore, to the person, normal. If the tension leads, in time, to pain, the person is more likely to say, "I have a bad back" than "My back hurts because of the chronic tension I've been putting on it." Some people are very tense, yet they insist that they are "relaxed" and "free." Only when they learn a better way and have some basis for comparison will they be able to recognize the tension and stiffness inherent in their old ways of moving.

❧

RECOVERING BALANCE

As pianists, our goal is to sit in balance so as to eliminate tension and have maximum freedom for our arms. However, balance in sitting is exactly like balance in standing, except that when we sit, the torso is supported by the bench, not by the legs. Therefore, we cannot cultivate balance just in sitting; we must cultivate it first in standing, then apply what we learn to sitting at the piano.

I shall discuss six pivotal areas of the body whose cooperative alignment produces easy uprightness. They are the "places of balance" listed below and shown in the illustration.

- The head on the spine at the AO joint
- The balance of the arm structure (shoulder joint)
- The lumbar spine
- The hip joint
- The knee joint
- The ankle joint

The vertical line in the drawing is an imaginary axis showing the relationship of the places of balance. The line illustrates the direction and organization of weight delivery through the bony structure. The key to recovering balance lies in understanding this organization and then Mapping it in one's own body. Notice that in the previous chapter, "Mapping the Structure," we described principal structures, such as "the skull," "the pelvis," or "the foot." In this chapter, by contrast, we speak of joints, not structures: "the AO joint," "the hip joint," "the ankle joint." This different way of speaking is intended to help develop a dynamic sense of the parts in relation to each other. Thinking of joints is the best way to do this, partly because kinesthetic receptors are concentrated in the joints.

The line in the illustration might suggest that we should always stand like the model in the picture. That is not its intent. If I stand still, in line at the bank, I may stand as in the picture. But as I move and perform different actions I will continually depart from balance and return to it. Balance is not a stance or position but a means of organizing movement, a place of reference, that place from which movement in any direction is easiest.

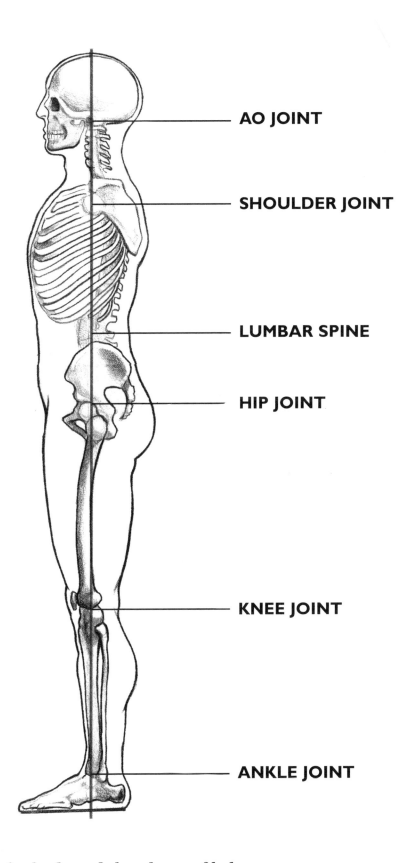

AO JOINT

SHOULDER JOINT

LUMBAR SPINE

HIP JOINT

KNEE JOINT

ANKLE JOINT

The core of the body and the places of balance.

THE HEAD ON THE SPINE: THE AO JOINT

The head rests more or less level on the top vertebra of the spine. The joint between the head and the spine is called the *atlanto-occipital* joint because it connects the *atlas*, the top vertebra of the spine, and the *occiput,* which is the lowest bone of the skull. Unfortunately, there is no common name for this joint in English, so I shall use the abbreviation "AO joint."

The top two vertebrae have special structural modifications to permit easy movement of the skull up and down (nodding) and side to side (shaking the head) without disturbing the balance. Remember that the jaw, which hangs from the skull, is not part of the skull. The head itself, without the jaw, is what we learn to balance. We allow the skull to find its natural relationship to the spine. In considering whether the skull is level, think of an imaginary line going straight back from the upper teeth to the bottom of the ears and on to the base of the skull.

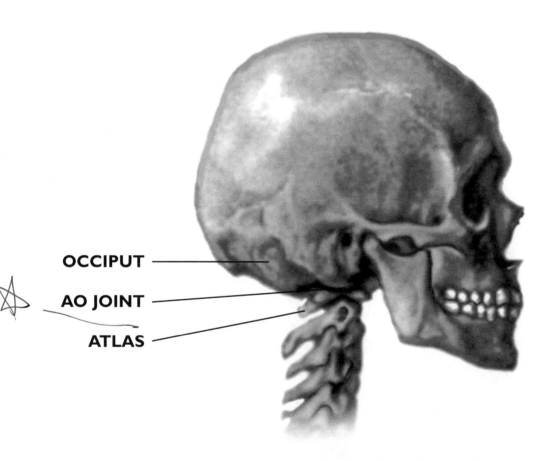

OCCIPUT

AO JOINT

ATLAS

The head rests in balance on the AO joint.

Become aware of your ears as the center, front to back, of the skull. Next, imagine a line through your head connecting your ears to each other. As you nod your head, you can be aware of the line connecting your ears as the axis of the nodding movement and notice that your spine does not need to move with your head. You can develop awareness of the AO joint. Locate it by pointing a finger directly at the back of your mouth. You are pointing to the AO joint (when doctors need an X-ray of the AO joint they point the X-ray machine at the back of the mouth just as you are pointing with your finger). Develop a vivid awareness of the location of the AO joint. There are numerous kinesthetic receptors in the AO joint to tell you about the head's movement.

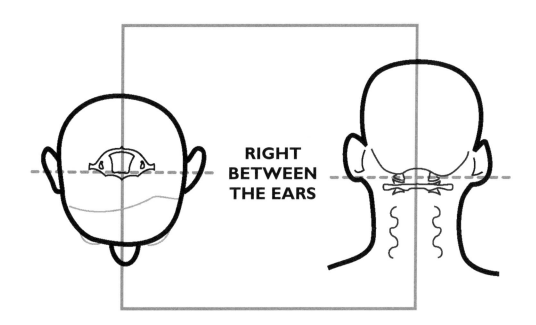

The AO joint is right between the ears,
both side to side and front to back.

Most of us have some tension in our necks. It was F. M. Alexander who recognized the harm done by tension in the neck and explained why improving our use of the rest of our bodies depends on releasing tension in the neck. The following thought experiment may help show why keeping the neck free is so important.

Imagine a length of broomstick about ten inches long with a small pumpkin attached to one end (the whole thing looks like half a dumbbell). The pumpkin is heavy— let's suppose it weighs ten pounds, about the weight of a head. Now stand the broomstick upright on a table with the pumpkin balanced on top of it, and hold the broomstick with one hand. If the broomstick is vertical, the pumpkin is balanced, and a small amount of force from your hand is enough to keep it upright. But suppose the broomstick tilts by forty-five degrees. In that position your hand must work hard to keep it from falling further.

Your head weighs about as much as the pumpkin. If your head is off balance, your neck muscles have to do about as much work to keep it from falling as your hand did to keep the pumpkin from falling. We have strong muscles in our necks.

They have to be massive and strong to move our heavy heads around. If the head, like our tilted pumpkin, is chronically off balance, those muscles have to be chronically tight. We may not notice the tension because we're accustomed to it, but our neck muscles are obliged to work all the time.

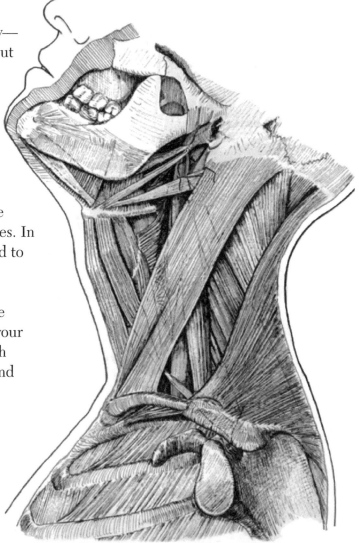

When neck muscles are free the head can tilt and turn while remaining balanced. Tense neck muscles generate tension elsewhere in the body.

FREE   **TIGHT**

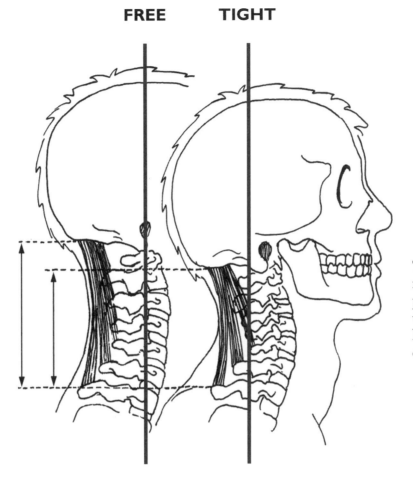

Free neck muscles permit easy movement of the head and the arms.

Tense neck muscles put pressure on the nerve-housing half of the spine.

Tension in the neck is a serious issue because it influences the whole body, but two facts about it are especially significant for pianists. First, some neck muscles attach to parts of the arm structure, and therefore, tense neck muscles inhibit the use of the arms. Second, the nerves that supply our arms branch off the spinal column in the neck region. Tense muscles in the neck can put pressure on those nerves, impairing the nerve supply to our arms and hands.

We learned earlier that imbalance of the head on the spine, besides causing neck muscles to tense, generates compensations elsewhere in the body. We can't get rid of the compensations unless we get rid of what they are compensations for—namely, imbalance of the head. So developing a freely balanced head and releasing tension in the neck are crucial for recovering overall balance and free motion throughout the body.

To free the neck it is vital to map it correctly. (It may be that mismapping the neck is a major cause of the neck tension that drags us off balance in the first place.) You can palpate the different superficial muscles of your neck. Lie down on the floor and massage your neck gently, discovering its structure and encouraging release. Alexander teachers frequently point out that a daily routine of this kind, which they call "constructive rest," can, over time, bring about tremendous improvement.

THE BALANCE OF THE ARM STRUCTURE: THE SHOULDER JOINT

Our arms do not support our weight when we stand or sit. But it is useful, especially for pianists, to include the shoulder joint among the places of balance. When balanced, the shoulder joint seen from the side (as in the illustration of the places of balance) is in the same vertical plane as the point of balance of the head on the spine (AO joint). The socket of the shoulder joint (glenoid fossa of the scapula) faces directly out to the side of the body, like another ear. When in balance, the arm structure is centered in relation to the ribs, giving maximum freedom to the arms, which is important for pianists. I discuss balance of the arm structure in detail in the chapter on the arm and hand, and support for the arms in the chapter on muscles.

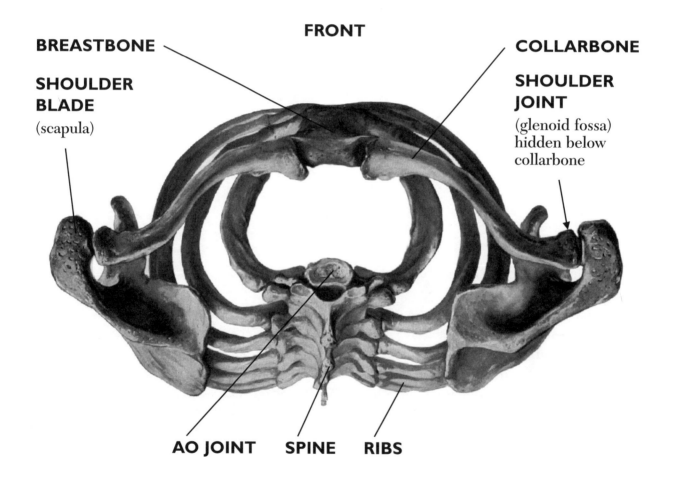

FRONT

BREASTBONE

SHOULDER BLADE
(scapula)

COLLARBONE

SHOULDER JOINT
(glenoid fossa) hidden below collarbone

AO JOINT   **SPINE**   **RIBS**

BACK

The collarbone and shoulder blade from above. Notice that the structure is balanced over the ribs in such a way that it centers over the weight-bearing part of the spine.

THE LUMBAR SPINE

Since the spine is curved, not all parts of it coincide with the vertical line connecting the places of balance in the illustration. But the lumbar portion of the spine does coincide with that line. The lumbar area is in the center of the body, front to back as well as side to side. When we are in balance it is directly below the place of balance of the head on the spine. We can become kinesthetically sensitive to these places of balance so that our balanced head and our lumbar spine and the relationship between them become objects of our awareness. This awareness can be the basis of a new sense of free movement organized around and emanating from support at our core.

Here is a way to develop awareness of your lumbar spine. Find the iliac crests of your pelvis, the curving top ridges of both pelvic bones. Place one thumb on the top of each iliac crest (see illustration, p. 45), and imagine a line through your body connecting your two thumbs to each other. The center of that line coincides with your lumbar spine. Taking a few steps backwards may enhance your awareness of it, for if your thorax has been thrust back it will automatically adjust forward over your lumbar vertebrae. Stay mindful of your head, at its place of balance between your ears, poised over the lumbar spine. Become aware of the whole spine as a curving column of support up the center of your body. Over time, you can develop increasing kinesthetic awareness of the AO joint in relation to the lumbar spine.

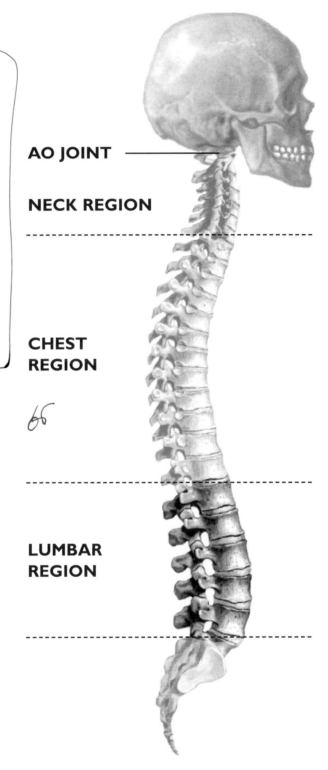

AO JOINT

NECK REGION

CHEST REGION

LUMBAR REGION

The head is balanced on the AO joint, directly above the lumbar region of the spine. The massive vertebrae of the lumbar region curve forward to a central position in the torso.

The curves of the spine permit it to absorb impact. Notice, though, that the curves occur naturally by themselves—we don't "do" them. In particular, the curve of the lumbar spine is not the result of any activity on our part but rather of the way vertebrae naturally relate to each other at rest. Any habit of "arching" the back is likely to be over-arching, which strains the lower back. Gripping and tensing—over-arching—the lower back are very common among pianists. A pianist who has been accustomed to over-arching or gripping the lower back may feel "slumped" at first when brought to balance. In such cases, a mirror is helpful to verify that what feels slumped is in fact upright.

***

❧

The tendency among organists is just the opposite. Because the feet are not firmly planted on the floor and because organists must often play on more than one keyboard, the tendency is to round the lumbar spine and rock back onto the tailbone.

***

❧

THE HIP JOINT

The hip joint is the middle, top to bottom, of the body. (If you think of your "waist" as your "middle," you should revise your body map.) When we stand in balance, the hip joint is aligned vertically with other places of balance: the AO joint, the shoulder joint, and the lumbar spine (see illustration of places of balance, p. 37). The hip joint is one of the most mobile joints of the body. Its "ball and socket" design permits three kinds of motion. We can move our legs forward and back (flexing and extending) as well as out to the side and back in (abducting and adducting). We can also rotate the leg at the hip joint.

The hip joint is lower than most people imagine. With your thumbs again on the iliac crest of your pelvis, reach down with your middle fingers about as far as you can. Take a couple of steps and you will feel a bone moving under your middle fingers. That is the greater trochanter, which is the top of the shaft of your femur. The hip joint is slightly higher than the greater trochanter. The hip joint is not only lower, it is further out to the side than many people imagine. The hip joint has a wealth of kinesthetic receptors to give information about its position and movement.

When you stand in balance, with the hip joint lined up with the other places of balance, you can release the muscles in your butt, which should not be tense when you are standing. "Tuck in your butt!" is one of the Posture Myths, and it is very bad advice. If you have a habit of tensing or tucking your butt, you are likely also to have a habit of rotating your entire leg slightly outward (so that your toes point out to the sides). This will cause the outside of the heels of your shoes to wear faster than the insides, and it is such a common habit that some manufacturers compensate for it by providing reinforcement on the outsides of the heels of their shoes. If the outsides of the heels of your shoes are much more heavily worn than the insides, that suggests that you need to pay attention to releasing the muscles of your butt. The release of your butt muscles will permit a slight inward rotation of your legs as they return to neutral. This release is vital for security and ease in sitting at the piano.

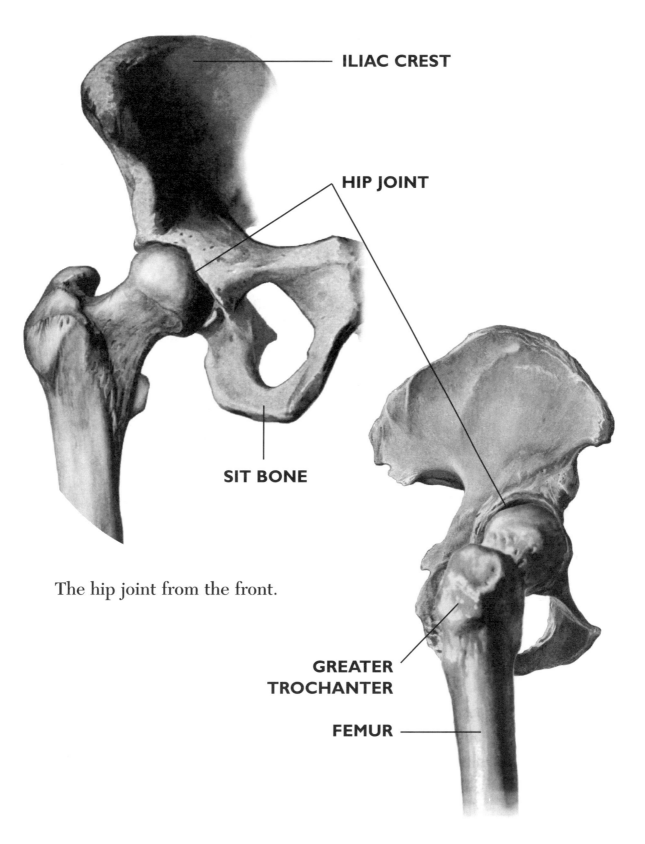

ILIAC CREST

HIP JOINT

SIT BONE

The hip joint from the front.

GREATER TROCHANTER

FEMUR

The hip joint from the side.

Sitting: The balance of the upper torso over the pelvis is the same whether we are standing or sitting. When we stand in balance the weight of the torso is delivered through the hip joints to the thighbones (femurs), which deliver it through the legs to the ground. When we sit, we bend at the hip joints, knees, and ankles, which causes the thighbones to move out of the way. The upper torso remains balanced over the pelvis with weight delivered through the sit bones to the bench.

The sit bones (ischeal tuberosities) are the lowest part of the pelvis. Because they are normally rounded, like the rockers on a rocking chair, some people call them "rockers." The rounded shape permits easy rocking motion of the pelvis forward and back. A few people have sit bones that are pointed instead of round, which makes rocking forward and back on the sit bones painful. Those people need a cushion to sit comfortably at the piano.

Since the sit bones are the lowest part of the pelvis, they are below the hip joints. Therefore, when the legs are fully bent at the

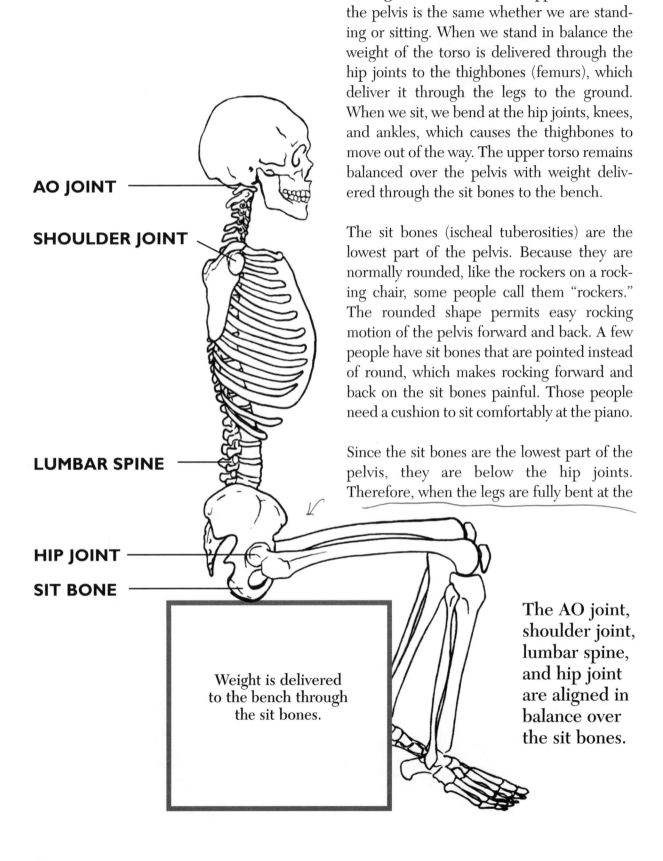

AO JOINT

SHOULDER JOINT

LUMBAR SPINE

HIP JOINT

SIT BONE

Weight is delivered to the bench through the sit bones.

The AO joint, shoulder joint, lumbar spine, and hip joint are aligned in balance over the sit bones.

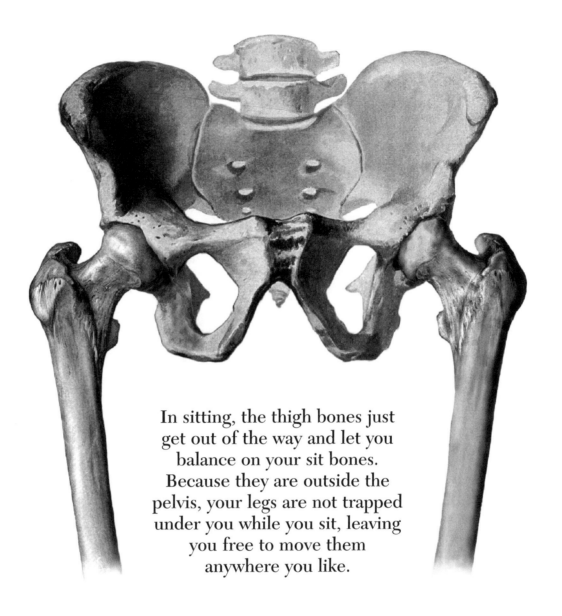

In sitting, the thigh bones just get out of the way and let you balance on your sit bones. Because they are outside the pelvis, your legs are not trapped under you while you sit, leaving you free to move them anywhere you like.

hip joints in sitting, the thighbones are *above* the sit bones. This permits the weight of the torso to be delivered through the sit bones to the bench, with none of the weight delivered to the legs. We sit on our sit bones, not on our legs. With weight properly delivered to the sit bones, the legs are free to move. We can use them for support as we play in different parts of the keyboard. We can put them in front of the bench, under the bench, out to the side, wherever we like. And, of course, we use our legs and feet to pedal. All these

movements should feel easy and should not confer any sense of instability. However, if a person sits so that weight is delivered to the back of the thigh instead of the sit bones, or thrown back toward the tailbone, movement will not be so easy. Sitting will be less comfortable, the legs will have limited mobility, the pedal may be hard to reach, and playing will be more difficult and less secure.

The release of tense butt muscles is vital for sitting. Tense butt muscles cause a slight outward rotation of the leg. When we sit, we must release any tense butt muscles, permitting legs to rotate inward, back to neutral. If this release does not occur, weight may be delivered to the back of the legs instead of to the sit bones.

There are thus two sorts of motion at the hip joint that make proper sitting possible. The first and most obvious is the bending motion that puts the thighbone at a right angle to the torso. The second is the release of any muscular tension that causes outward rotation of the leg.

As you sit, feel the muscles of your butt "fan" outward from the sacrum, so that the heads of your thighbones feel out to the sides of your pelvis and higher than your sit bones. You can develop awareness of the sit bones delivering weight to the bench, which leaves your legs free to move.

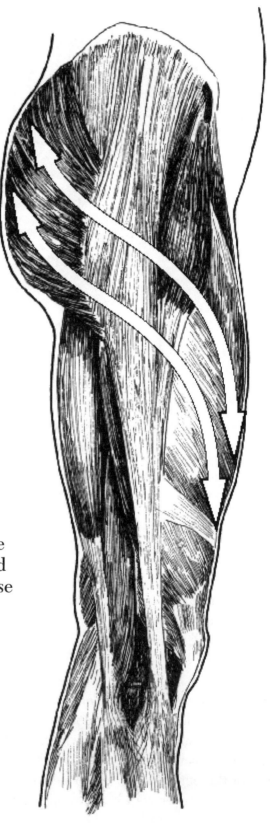

These muscles fan out from the sacrum. They are shortened and narrowed by tension, so as you free them they lengthen and widen, and your lower back regains a nice sense of roundness.

This release will feel like a downward drop of the butt, not to be confused with tucking the butt.

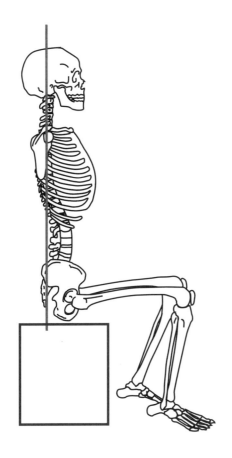

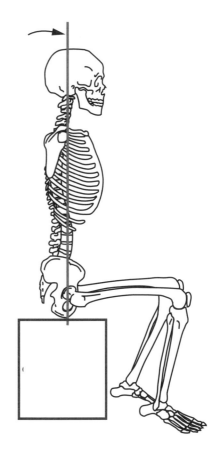

Back-oriented sitting.

**Weight is thrown back toward the
nerve half of the spine.**

Balanced sitting.

**Weight is centered over the
hip joints and sit bones.**

If the hip joints do not bend far enough, the pelvis will tilt backwards, throwing the weight toward the tailbone (which can't bear it) and forcing arm and torso muscles to compensate. This is *back-oriented* sitting. It results in tension in the arms and back as well as potential back, shoulder, and arm pain. Insufficient bending of the hip joints may also cause weight to be delivered to the backs of the thighs instead of to the sit bones.

Many pianists, perhaps the majority, sit in back-oriented fashion. The weight is thrown backwards and the pianist has to compensate

for the imbalance by tensing torso and arm muscles. The playing suffers. Back orientation has several causes. The pianist may have mismapped the spine and may imagine that support for the upper body comes from the surface of the back instead of from the core (remember the spine-back distinction). Back orientation can result from insufficient bending at the hip joint, which leaves the pelvis tilted backwards, throwing the weight to the rear, toward the tailbone (which can't bear weight). Back orientation can also come from the Posture Myths. If a person's concept of sitting up straight includes "shoulders back, chest out" and the rest of that dreadful catechism, the person is likely to arch the lower back and stiffen the shoulder area. This is extremely common among pianists. So is back and shoulder pain.

Pianists need to be sure that the hip joint is sufficiently bent so that the pelvis is not tilted backward, and that the lower back is released (which if you have been gripping or over-arching will feel like letting it fall outwards). For someone who has been back oriented, the balanced alignment of the upper torso will be forward of what the person has been accustomed to. When brought to balance, people who have been back oriented typically feel that they are slumped forwards. If someone feels slumped forwards when brought to balance, the best thing to do is to look in a mirror and verify that what feels slumped (because the habitual tension is gone) is really upright. It is also worthwhile to truly slump forwards in front of the mirror so as to be clear about the difference. To someone who has been chronically back oriented or chronically slumped, being upright and in balance may feel like cheating—sitting isn't supposed to be that easy.

Pay attention and develop awareness of the relationship between your AO joint, your lumbar spine, and your hip joints. When they are aligned vertically you can release muscles on the back and the front of your torso. This helps to free your arms; it also helps you develop awareness of your central core support.

Sitting in balance on the sit bones gives both stability and mobility, enabling a pianist to move side to side, forward and back, and spiral, as required by the music, without loss of freedom. In these movements, the head leads, the entire spine moves (remember the

Laws of the Spine), and the pelvis moves in relation to the legs. That is, the pianist moves freely at the hip joint with a movement that includes the whole spine. Unfortunately, many pianists plant the pelvis on the bench and then move exclusively from the waist. That is *not* a good idea. Remember: the "waist" is a colloquially designated region of the body that is of interest mainly to clothing manufacturers and dieters. It is not an anatomical structure; most important, it is not a joint. Awareness of the entire length of the torso from AO joint to pelvis organizes movement and gives freedom.

Pianists need to be aware that the pelvis is the lower part of the upper body, not the upper part of the lower body. Therefore, when we sit on the piano bench, our *entire* upper body is on the bench. We need to map the pelvis as *part* of the upper body. We should not think of it as a base or foundation above which the upper body moves.

Some people map the hip joint as the place where leg motion occurs, but not the place where torso motion occurs. As a result, they may bend at the hip joint to sit down, but then while sitting they bend from the waist instead of the hip joint to play in different parts of the keyboard. They may bend at the hip joint to sit, but when the performance is over they bend at the waist to take a bow. These people need to understand and to feel that leg movements and torso movements both originate at the hip joint.

All too often, when pianists adjust sideways they initiate with the shoulder or the chest instead of leading with the head. The appearance is of the shoulder being thrust sideways and the lower back and head staying behind.

It looks angular and compressed. By contrast, when the head leads, a movement results which may look like a long, easy **C** curve of the spine that is fluid and graceful. Subjectively, these movements are night and day, the one interfering with the arms, the other supporting them. Again, remember the Laws of the Spine. Once a person learns to lead with the head, the amount of sideways movement needed to reach the extremes of the piano will seem smaller than before, as if the keyboard had shrunk. The correct movement, with the head leading, feels both *smaller* and *more secure.*

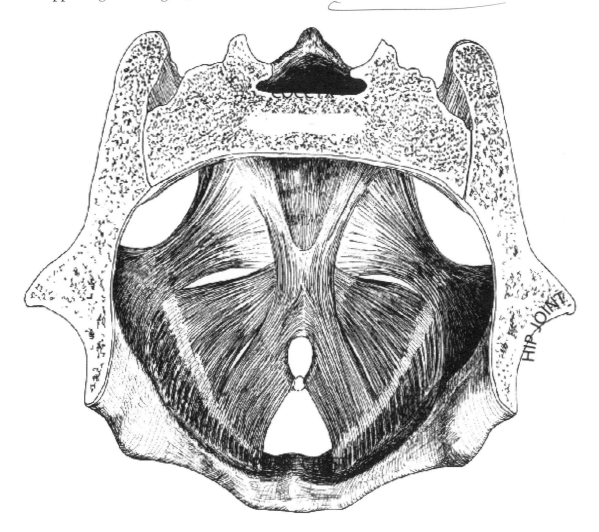

Muscles of the pelvic floor.

Release of the muscles of the pelvic floor is also essential. The muscular "floor" of the pelvis supports the internal organs, and it moves automatically as we breathe. Habits of gripping in the lower back, or in the quadri- ceps, or mismapping the movements of pedal- ing may, any of them, cause the muscles of the pelvic floor to tighten, inhibiting breathing and interfering with a pianist's sense of contact and support from the bench. The proper feeling of being "grounded" on the sit bones requires that the pelvic floor be released.

Feel that you release the inside of your pelvis. The sensation may be of releasing directly downward onto the bench; one student described it as "puddling down." Notice the accompanying release of the quadriceps muscles in the thigh. Without tightening the pelvic floor, notice that you can move side to side, forward and back (bending, of course, at the hip joint), while retaining the sense of goundedness on the bench. When you do this, your arms move more freely also. The sensation is that letting go the pelvic floor allows the arms to "float." (See "Suspension of the Arms" in Chapter 5.)

❧

For organists the importance of understanding how to sit has further implications. Back orientation is bad enough if and when the feet are planted on the floor and providing support. But organists use the lower part of their bodies (from the hip joint to the feet) for playing. When organists sit back on the tailbone in a back-oriented position, several things happen. There is an inevitable rounding of the spine and a corresponding loss of the balance of the head on the AO joint. Because the feet are not providing support, this places enormous strain on the muscles of the neck and back. There is also a severe loss of mobility in the legs and feet, mobility that must be available to develop a good pedal technique. The arm structure is also thrown out of balance, severely limiting the ability to play freely and to reach upper keyboards and stops. Organists who first become aware of their back orientation and attempt to correct it often complain that they are going to fall forward and off the bench. (This never actually happens.) The "cure" for this most common of organists' maladies is first to find the proper place of balance on the sit bones, and to learn how to move in and out of that balance. An additional challenge for organists comes from not being able to have the feet firmly planted on the floor at all times. As a result, there are many times when some of the weight of the legs must be transferred UPWARD into the hip joint and then into the sit bones. In order to do this the muscles of the upper leg, buttocks, and groin area must be activated and available in the way they would be if you were about to stand up.

Sitting on the organ bench, place your hands on the sides of the lower keyboard and rock from side to side, then back and forth. As you do, locate the sit bones. As you develop this awareness, experiment with finding your hip joints and become aware of the mobility you have in your legs. This will require activating the muscles of the upper leg, groin, and buttocks. Reach for the upper and lower parts of the pedalboard while rocking on your sit bones. This kind of creative playing around, combined with a correct body map, will certainly lead to improved movement.

Going from Standing to Sitting: Sometimes a person will stand in balance but then destroy the balance in the act of sitting down. One thing that often goes wrong is that the person bends at the waist instead of at the hip joint. Remember, there is no joint called "the waist." People who think of the waist as the "middle" of the body are more likely to bend at the waist. (The middle of the body, top to bottom, is the hip joint.) Remember also that the act of sitting is not mainly a bending of the spine. It is mainly a bending of the hip joints, knee joints, and ankles.

As you sit down, retain awareness of the entire length of the spine, from the head to the pelvis, and of the relationship of the three places of balance: the AO joint, lumbar spine, and hip joints. Let your legs move out of the way by bending at the hip joints, knees, and ankles and place your sit bones, with the torso above them, on the chair.

ॐ

THE HEIGHT OF THE BENCH

Many piano methods include some discussion of bench height. They are likely to recommend something like this: "The forearm should be level when the student sits erect without hunching the shoulders," which is good advice (provided "erect" does not mean "in accordance with the Posture Myths"). Much the same advice is found in any ergonomics text. The optimum bench height is whatever height leaves the forearm level. It is not the same for everyone, and it may not be the same even for people of the same stature. The optimum bench height is determined by the ratio between the length of the arm and the length of the torso, and this ratio varies from one person to another.

To many pianists, the optimum height will feel high at first, since most benches are too low for most people. Even adjustable benches do not go high enough for many people.

If a person sits at a height that is not optimal, some adaptation to the less advantageous height will be required. Adaptations that involve tension can lead to problems. A person sitting too low may hunch the shoulders or lift the elbows or clench the fingers as if to grab the piano to compensate for a feeling of the hands falling off the keyboard. A person sitting too high may drop the wrist or pull the collarbone and shoulder blade down. All of these compensations involve static muscular activity—tension—that limits freedom and can in time lead to injury.

A handy way to find the optimum height is to compare the tip of the elbow with the top of the white keys. That is: when you sit in balance with your fingertips on the keys, in playing position in the mid-range of the keyboard, the tip of your elbow should be about on the same plane as the top of the white keys. To determine whether the bench height is optimum you will at first need a mirror or a friend to observe you (there is no way to twist yourself around to see). Once you become accustomed to playing at the optimum height your kinesthetic sense will tell you, the moment you sit down, whether the height is right. If the height is wrong, you'll do whatever you need to do to correct it since you will also know (again, thanks to your newly-sensitive kinesthetic sense) how much more difficult it is to play when sitting too low or too high.

Adjustable benches are a perfect way to control the height of the bench. Their only drawback is their high cost. Before buying one, make sure it will go high enough for you and anyone else who may use it. Many adjustable benches, particularly the expensive "artists' benches," do not go high enough for many people. Mine does not go high enough for me, so I set it on two lengths of 2″ x 8″ boards to bring it to the proper height. That is a good solution, better than sitting on cushions or Beethoven Sonatas, although the boards are a nuisance to remove for others who do not need them. Carpet samples, available free or at low cost from a carpet store, are an excellent way to adjust the height of the bench. They provide better support for sitting than cushions. If you are a teacher and do not have an adjustable bench, you can get a supply of carpet samples and each student will quickly learn to put the appropriate number of carpet squares on the bench at the start of the lesson. Make sure they have carpet squares, or some other solution, at home also.

Some pianists and teachers pay scant attention to the height of the bench, which surprises me since it is such an easy correction to make. I suspect one reason is that they have not experienced the difference optimal bench height makes in their own playing or their students' playing. The most convincing demonstration I know is this: listen to a pianist or student who is accustomed to sitting at a disadvantageous height. Then put the student at the optimum height and listen again. In almost every case there will be an immediate improvement in the playing.

A bench height that is not optimum will not necessarily cause injury; pianists who know how to move without tension can play with the bench higher or lower and not be injured (as organists must do when they play different manuals, or some keyboard players do when they play standing up). The reason to adopt the optimal bench height is not to avoid injury but to make playing easier. The optimal height gives us the greatest mechanical advantage in relation to the piano, so piano playing requires less work. No pianist I know who has become accustomed to the greater ease that the optimal height affords has the slightest inclination to change back.

For organists the issue of proper bench height is even more complicated. The proper bench height cannot be determined from the relation of the elbow to the keyboard because most organs have at least two keyboards, and often three or even four or five. If we assume that the torso is properly balanced on the sit bones, most organists will be able to move from one keyboard to another by gently rocking forward or backward on the sit bones while still maintaining proper balance and a sense of freedom of movement. Rocking forward on the sit bones to reach an upper keyboard feels very much like the movement one makes while preparing to stand up. This rocking forward movement should be practiced until it becomes a natural part of your technique.

The critical measurement for organists is the distance between the top of the bench and the top of the pedal keys, and how this distance relates to the length of the tibia (shinbone). If one is using a toe-heel pedal technique, the bench should be high enough for the toes to rest very slightly on the pedals while the heels are just slightly above the key surface. For the all-toe technique often used in Baroque and early music, the bench should be slightly higher so the toes are comfortably touching the pedals and the heels are up and out of the way.

As with pianists, many organists sit too low. When sitting too low, most organists feel as though they need to hold their legs up and off the pedalboard. This forces the player to lean back onto the tailbone and causes the lumbar spine to round and the head to be pulled forward. This distortion of the balance of the torso makes it impossible for the legs to move freely, and tightens and inhibits the arm structure, making it difficult to move freely and to reach the keyboards. Those few organists who sit too high are likely to experience difficulty in moving the legs freely, over-arching of the lumbar spine, and, as with pianists, wrists that are too low. For persons who are either very tall or very short, there may need to be a compromise in the bench height between what is ideal for the legs and what is an ideal alignment with the main keyboard.

Another consideration is the distance of the bench from the organ console. Most organists play too close to the keyboards, which restricts movement of the arms and legs. Organists who sit too close often tense the arm structure and can sometimes be seen holding the elbows against their torso.

THE KNEE JOINT

Weight is delivered through the knee joint to the tibia or "shinbone." The shinbone is the more massive of the two bones in the lower leg (the other, smaller one is the fibula), and it is the one in front. It lies just below the skin in the front of the lower leg. You can palpate the shinbone along its entire length. When we stand in balance, the knee joint (as seen from the side) aligns directly below the hip joint. It is *lower than* the kneecap and *behind* it. Notice that the knee is not a "thing"—not a physical structure. It is a *joint*. The joint lies *between* two bones, the thighbone and the shinbone, and it is the place where those bones move relative to each other. Locating the joint precisely—Mapping it correctly—permits motion at the joint to be free.

Belief that the knee is a thing—a knob or a ball—is a common mismapping and it causes motion to be stiff. Once again, the knee is not a *thing*, it is a *joint*. Some people seem to think that the knee joint is directly behind the kneecap, instead of behind and below it. That mismapping creates a lot of tension. Often, people who mismap the knee joint that way have pain in walking, as well as difficult movement at the piano. If your legs feel tired or sore from long periods of standing, it may help if you accurately map your knee joint and cultivate awareness of weight delivery through the joint.

The only motion possible at the knee joint is bending and unbending (flexing and extending). We cannot abduct or adduct at the knee, nor can we rotate (rotation of the leg is a rotation of the entire leg, not just the lower leg, and it occurs at the hip joint, not the knee joint).

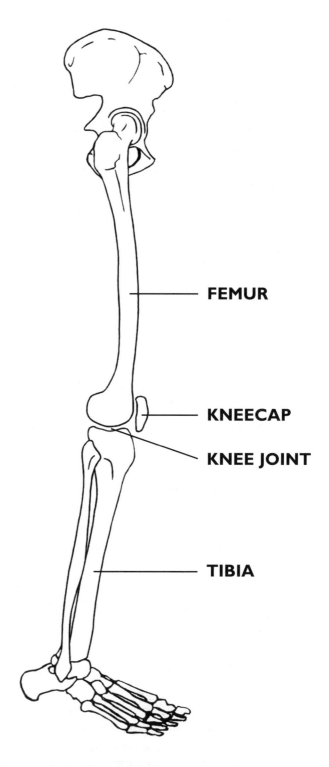

FEMUR

KNEECAP

KNEE JOINT

TIBIA

Knee joint behind and below the kneecap. Weight is delivered from the femur to the tibia (the front bone of the lower leg).

When standing, be aware of your knee joint, lower than the kneecap and posterior to it. Become aware of the knee joint lined up directly below the AO joint, lumbar spine, and hip joint. Then try for a moment to stand as if weight were delivered through the front of the knee (the kneecap). Having experienced that, notice what a difference it makes when you think, correctly, of weight delivered through the knee joint behind and below the kneecap, to the shinbone, the ankle joint, and the floor. Notice that at balance the knee does not "lock" nor does it bend. It also does not feel tense.

If a person is chronically off balance, the knees will chronically lock in order to stabilize the body and thereby reduce pressure on the discs of the lower back. Chronic locking of the knees is a compensation for imbalance of the torso. It is an issue for pianists because someone whose knees are chronically locked when standing will be off balance when sitting also. Attempting to unlock the knees without correcting the imbalance for which locked knees are a compensation will just make matters worse. The person must learn to balance the torso, which permits the knees to return to the unlocked, balanced position. Then the person can find balance sitting at the piano.

〜

THE ANKLE JOINT

Weight is delivered by the shinbone to the foot through the ankle joint, which is at the front of the heel bone.

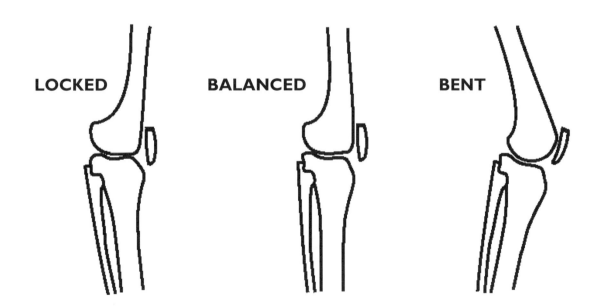

LOCKED   **BALANCED**   **BENT**

Bending occurs at the joint, not at the kneecap.

When you stand in balance you can be aware that your weight is delivered to the ankle joint, at the front of the heel bone. This permits a feeling of being "centered" over your feet. Some people imagine that weight is delivered to the back of their heel bone, as if their lower leg and foot were L-shaped with weight delivered to the corner of the L. Just for comparison, try standing that way. Notice how it throws your weight backward and triggers compensating tension throughout the body. Now return to balance with weight delivered to the ankle joint at the front end of the heel bone and notice the release. You should practice being aware of the ankle joint in vertical relationship with the other places

of balance—AO joint, shoulder joint, lumbar spine, hip joint, and knee joint.

Proper mapping of the ankle joint is vital for pedaling. Some pianists are surprised to learn that improper pedaling can cause problems, but approximately one pianist in twenty gets pain from pedaling because of mismapping the ankle joint. That sounds like a small number, but it means that if you are a teacher the odds are good that at least one of your students has this problem. Some students avoid using the pedal at home and pedal only at lessons. You need to ask your students if they have pain when they pedal. If they do, you need to address the mapping problem.

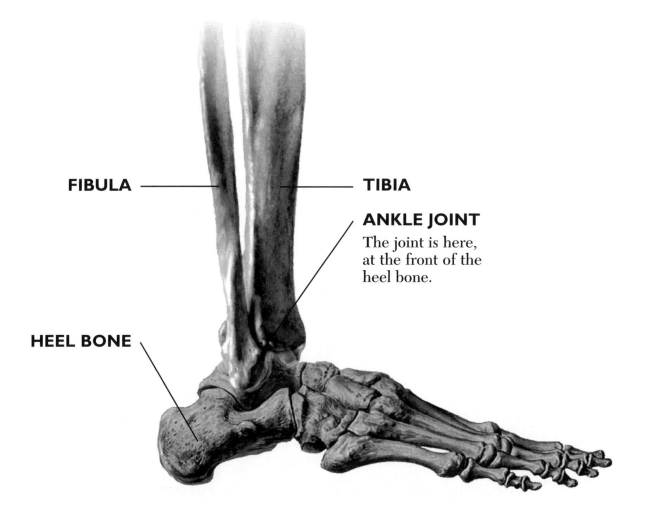

FIBULA

TIBIA

ANKLE JOINT
The joint is here, at the front of the heel bone.

HEEL BONE

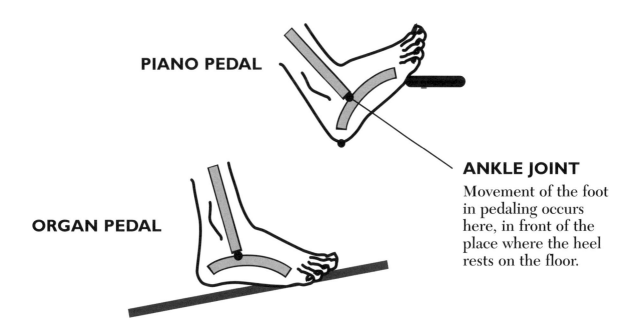

PIANO PEDAL

ORGAN PEDAL

ANKLE JOINT
Movement of the foot in pedaling occurs here, in front of the place where the heel rests on the floor.

The vital point here is that movement of the foot does not occur at the back of the heel bone, it occurs at the ankle joint which is in the *front* of the heel bone. In other words, our feet do not move like a capital letter **L** with a hinge at the corner:

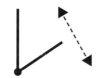

They move like a lopsided upside-down letter **T**:

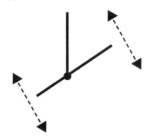

When you depress a piano pedal, the back of your heel does rest on the floor. But the movement of the foot is not there, where the heel touches the floor; it is in front of that, at the ankle joint. Mismapping this movement causes a predictable pattern of tension and pain: soreness in the shins, tension in the quadriceps muscles (the front of the thigh), and over-arching of the lower back. If our feet were **L**-shaped, with the movement at the back of the heel bone, then we could rest our heels on the floor and move only our foot. This is what the person who maps the foot as an **L** may try to do, with tension as the result.

But in fact we cannot move only our foot when we pedal. Since the joint is at the front of the heel bone and the pivot is at the back of the heel bone where it rests on the floor, moving the foot up and down to pedal will necessarily involve some up-and-down movement of the ankle joint itself, and consequently of the rest of the leg. This up-and-down movement of the leg means that pedaling involves movement not only at the ankle joint, but small movements of the knee and hip joints as well.

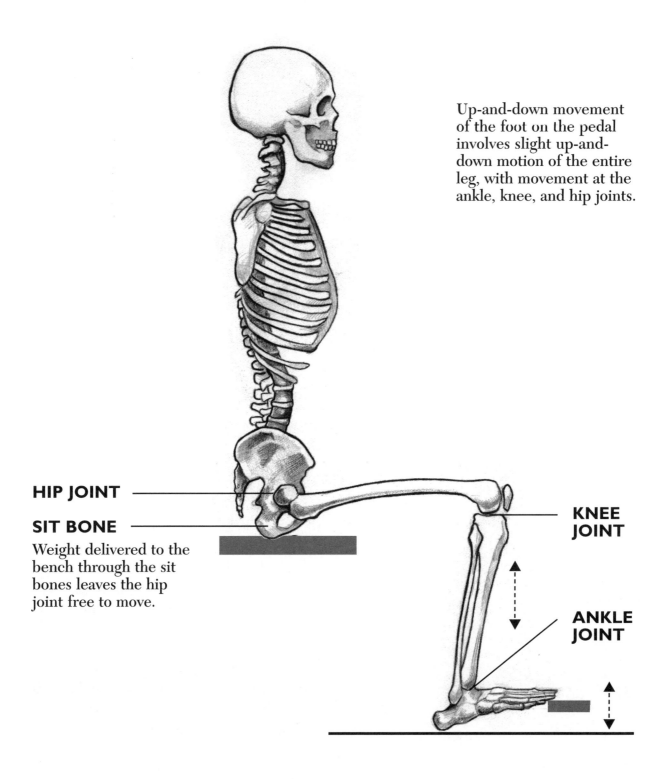

Up-and-down movement of the foot on the pedal involves slight up-and-down motion of the entire leg, with movement at the ankle, knee, and hip joints.

HIP JOINT

SIT BONE

Weight delivered to the bench through the sit bones leaves the hip joint free to move.

KNEE JOINT

ANKLE JOINT

The small movements of the knee and hip joints in pedaling provide further insight into the importance of sitting in balance. If a person sits with weight properly delivered to the sit bones, the legs are free to move. But if a person sits improperly, either with weight thrown backwards or with weight on the back of the thighs instead of on the sit bones, the movement of pedaling will cause instability which will have to be compensated by tensing. When we sit in balance and move the ankle joint correctly, pedaling is easy; it requires no compensating tension and does not disturb the balance of the torso.

Proper mapping of the ankle joint is vital for organists as well as pianists. Organists manipulate expression pedals using very much the same movement pianists use while pedaling (flexion and extension), as well as a side-to-side movement. More importantly, however, organists must move the ankle in virtually all directions to obtain a fluid and proficient pedal technique.

Sit at the console and play a chromatic scale on the pedalboard using a toe-heel technique. Become aware of the fact that the ankle joint is not located at the back of the L shape, but rather further forward. This understanding will enable free movement of both the toes and heels. Practice also opening and closing the swell box or crescendo pedal, being aware of the movement the ankle makes and where that movement occurs.

MAPPING THE INTERRELATION OF THE PLACES OF BALANCE

This chapter has described the structure and movement of each of the places of balance, and every pianist should thoroughly assimilate the information. But the places of balance do not function separately from each other in organizing our movement. All of them work together to organize our movement. That is, we do not just move our head on the spine or our legs at the hip joint, though we may focus on those places as we cultivate kinesthetic awareness. In the end, we move our bodies, not just the individual parts. When we move well, we exhibit freedom and fluidity throughout the body; awareness of the interrelation of the places of balance helps us to achieve this.

Turn back to the illustration of the places of balance on page 37. That is one of the most important illustrations in this book. You should make photocopies of it and post them everywhere in your house. Use them to remind yourself to focus attention on the places of balance and their relation to each other. Try to see the illustration not as an example of static "posture;" think of it potentially in motion: it exhibits the organization from which movement in any direction is easiest. Develop growing kinesthetic awareness of each place of balance. You might, for example, choose a different one each day as your focus. In time you will develop awareness of movement organized around the places of balance as you walk, stand, sit, and play the piano.

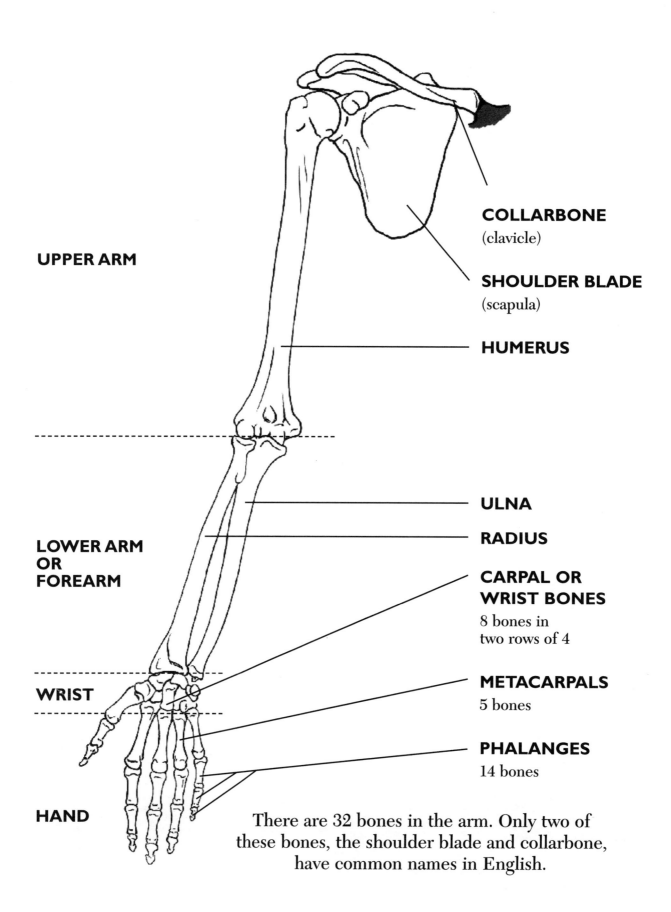

UPPER ARM

COLLARBONE
(clavicle)

SHOULDER BLADE
(scapula)

HUMERUS

ULNA

RADIUS

**LOWER ARM
OR
FOREARM**

**CARPAL OR
WRIST BONES**
8 bones in
two rows of 4

METACARPALS
5 bones

WRIST

PHALANGES
14 bones

HAND

There are 32 bones in the arm. Only two of
these bones, the shoulder blade and collarbone,
have common names in English.

CHAPTER 4: MAPPING THE ARM AND HAND

✌ THE WHOLE ARM

Unlike the forelimbs of other vertebrates, our arms play no weight-bearing role in locomotion and are free to function primarily as manipulating structures. The range of tasks they perform is truly astonishing, but it carries risks. One authority describes the arm as "an amazingly versatile unit that allows a wide range of movement, is exceptionally strong for its size, is capable of the most delicate and precise manipulation, and alternately, is strong enough to damage itself" (Putz-Anderson, p. 9). The neurologist Frank R. Wilson writes that "From the perspective of *biomechanical* anatomy, the hand is an integral part of the entire arm, a specialized termination of a cranelike structure suspended from the neck and upper chest" (*The Hand*, p. 8).

It is vital for pianists to develop a vivid kinesthetic awareness of the whole arm, and to map the shoulder blade and collarbone as part of the arm. The shoulder blade and collarbone do not connect to the ribs, nor do they rest on the ribs. The arm structure attaches to the rest of the skeleton in only one place, the sternoclavicular joint, where the collarbone meets the breastbone. When the arms are in balance, the shoulder blades can move freely over the ribs.

The outer end of the collarbone is attached to the shoulder blade by a joint and by very strong ligaments that prevent the shoulder blade and collarbone from moving relative to each other: when one moves, the other moves. Consequently, when we move our shoulder blade, the collarbone moves also. The movement of the collarbone and shoulder blade occurs at the sternoclavicular joint.

In piano playing, movements of the shoulder blade and collarbone are usually small, but they are absolutely vital for free playing (and for avoiding back and shoulder pain). The movements may be small, but if you have had a habit of fixing the shoulder blade and collarbone (as many pianists do), they will feel large at first. Also, if you were taught to hold your shoulders still, or if a teacher's demand that you not "hunch" your shoulders caused a habit of pulling them down, the proper movements will not only feel large, they will feel like cheating—forbidden pleasures. Give yourself permission to enjoy them.

Many pianists think that their arms end at the shoulder joint. That is, their body maps include a "shoulder-arm split" according to which the shoulder is part of the body, and the arm is separate from the body. One consequence of the shoulder-arm split is the fixing of the collarbone and shoulder blade, which is bad for several reasons. First, if the shoulder blade and collarbone are fixed, they will not contribute their share of movement

SHOULDER BLADE MOVEMENTS

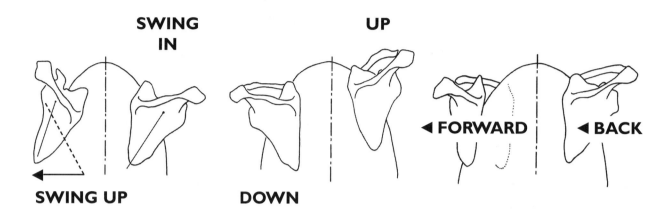

The shoulder blades can move in myriad ways: swinging down and up, moving in and out, forward and back, rotating over the ribs. Pianists should consciously develop awareness of the mobility of the shoulder blades.

and the rest of the arm must work harder. Some movements (such as crossing one hand in front of the body) become more difficult and less secure. Second, the fixing of the shoulder blade and collarbone actually inhibit movement of the upper arm, making movement stiffer and requiring more work. That is because the muscles used to fix the shoulder blade and collarbone also affect the movement of the humerus. Third, fixing the shoulder blade and collarbone often leads to back, shoulder, and neck pain.

Another consequence of the shoulder-arm split is that although motion of the shoulder blade and collarbone occur, they occur too late. It may help to bear in mind that the numerous bodily movements that facilitate and enable the playing of each note are preparatory—they occur *before* playing the note.

The shoulder-arm split may result from thinking of the shoulder as a clearly defined part of the body different from the arm. Remember that the word "shoulder" does not name an anatomical structure. Like the word "waist," it is used colloquially to designate a region of the body. Our concept of "shoulder" is derived, perhaps, from seeing people in football uniforms whose padding produces grotesquely enlarged "shoulders." Or from looking at muscular individuals whose well-developed deltoid muscles seem to define a knob at the top of their arms. Or from women's dresses with shoulder pads. Whatever its origin, the fantasy of a shoulder as a distinct part of the body is a concept to get rid of, since it affects the way we move and therefore the way we play the piano. You can verify this as follows, alone or with a colleague or student.

Imagine your arms as appendages to a football uniform-like shoulder. Move them back and forth and out to the sides with that image in mind. Lift them as if to put your hands on the piano keyboard, always with the image that they are attached to but distinct from a well-developed "shoulder." Now, retaining that image, play a passage on the piano and notice how it feels.

Now contrast that feeling with the feeling you get when you think of your arms as unified structures connected in front to the sternum at the base of the neck. Swing your arms back and forth with this new conception in mind; lift them to the sides and lift them as if to a piano keyboard, always thinking of each arm as one structure comprised of units connected by joints from the sternum to the fingertips. Retaining this new understanding of the arms as unified, freely moving structures attached to the sternum at the base of your neck, play the same passage on the piano. Is the passage suddenly easier? Almost invariably it is.

A joint is a place where two or more bones come together, usually in such a way that motion is possible at the joint. The bones do not connect to each other directly; instead they are surrounded and held together by a layer of ligaments and cartilage called the joint capsule. The surface of

---

❧

Mismapping of the arm structure and the subsequent fixing of the collarbone and shoulder blade have additional implications for the organist. In order to reach freely to an upper keyboard, one must not only rock gently forward on the sit bones, but the collarbone and shoulder blades must be free to move as well. As you reach up for a higher keyboard, there will be slight movement in the sterno-clavicular joint as the shoulder blades move up and out in a sort of hugging or wrapping-around gesture.

It can be helpful for the organist to sit at the console and experiment with these movements without actually playing. Sit balanced on the sit bones, then rock slightly forward while extending the arms out and around as though hugging a tree. Then practice using this gesture to reach the upper keyboard, and finally to play on the upper keyboard. If the arm structure is free to move and there is no fixing of the collarbone and shoulder blade, the balance of the torso on the sit bones will be retained while at the same time enabling the hands to move freely to upper keyboards and to manipulate stops.

the bone where it comes together with another bone is the articular surface. The shape of the articular surface and the characteristics of the ligaments holding the bones together determine what kinds of motion are possible at each joint.

Just as a joint is a juxtaposition of bones, the name of a joint is a juxtaposition of names of bones. This is a perspicuous convention, although the language used is Latin, not English. Thus, the joint of the hand with the finger is the "metacarpophalangeal" joint because it connects the metacarpal (or "hand") bone to the phalanx (or "finger") bone. Similarly, the joint of the breastbone with the collarbone is the "sternoclavicular" joint because it connects the sternum (breastbone) to the clavicle (collarbone). Once you know the names of the bones, the names of the joints follow as a matter of course, with the bone closer to the center of the body being named first. Since many joints in the arm and hand have no unambiguous common names in English, I shall often be obliged to use the technical names.

All the joints of the arm and hand are used in free piano playing, so pianists need to accurately map the various joints and their movements. Many pianists' injuries and limitations are the result of mismapping the movements that occur at the various arm joints. Pianists need to develop a sense of the arm structure as a whole with four principal joints. Because the receptors of our kinesthetic sense are concentrated in our joints, a good habit for pianists to develop is to "think joints." Most pianists will profit from mapping the movements of the different joints and

allowing movement to involve the whole arm from the fingertips to the tip of the collarbone at the sternoclavicular joint. The sense that the whole arm, all four major joints, is the structure that is moving to permit ease in playing brings about a better distribution of movement among the various joints, with no part doing more or less than its share.

Some pianists regard joints as fixed, or stable, places to move from. The shoulder joint, for example, is sometimes called a fixed place from which the arm moves. But that way of talking can have bad and serious consequences. Thinking of one part of the body as a fixed place from which to move another part of the body generates tension. The only way my shoulder joint, or any other joint, can act as a fixed place to move from is by my fixing it—that is, by tensing muscles. If I think of my wrist as a stable place to move from, I will stabilize it by tensing my arm; if I think of my shoulder as a stable place to move from, I will tense my back and chest muscles. The problem is not solved, it is only papered over by shifting the vocabulary—calling the joints "fulcrums" instead of "joints" or using the word "stable" instead of "fixed."

Regarding joints as fixed places to move from is sometimes supported by a general assertion that any bodily motion requires a fixed or stable place to move from. But that is a mismapping of bodily motion. I can raise my hand above my head using a free, fluid motion that involves my hand, forearm, upper arm, collarbone, and shoulder blade, with a sense of support in my core and no part of my body acting as a fixed place to move from. When I move that way, I move

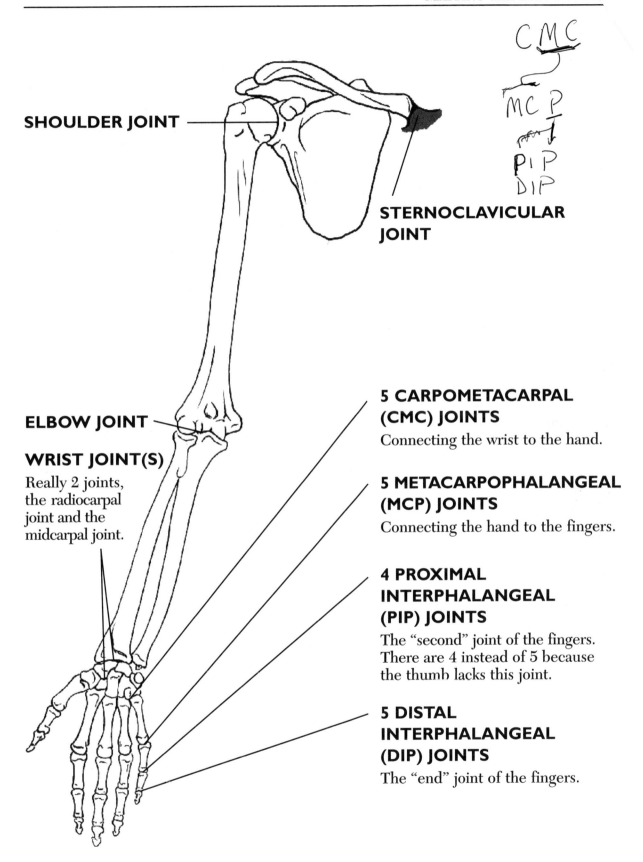

SHOULDER JOINT

STERNOCLAVICULAR JOINT

ELBOW JOINT

WRIST JOINT(S)

Really 2 joints, the radiocarpal joint and the midcarpal joint.

5 CARPOMETACARPAL (CMC) JOINTS

Connecting the wrist to the hand.

5 METACARPOPHALANGEAL (MCP) JOINTS

Connecting the hand to the fingers.

4 PROXIMAL INTERPHALANGEAL (PIP) JOINTS

The "second" joint of the fingers. There are 4 instead of 5 because the thumb lacks this joint.

5 DISTAL INTERPHALANGEAL (DIP) JOINTS

The "end" joint of the fingers.

The 32 bones of the arm are connected by 24 joints.

better than if I think of one part as a stable place to move from.

Nevertheless, there is another way in which it is essential for pianists to think of a fixed place to move from. That place, however, is not a body part; it is not inside our body at all. Instead, the fixed places we move from are the bench and the floor. Support from the bench and the floor, through our core support, permits us to move with ease and fluency, with no fixing of any part.

Many pianists are not aware of their whole arms as they play; their awareness extends at most from the fingers to the elbow and does not include the upper arm, shoulder blade, and collarbone. When the four arm joints are accurately mapped and free, the upper arm, including the collarbone and shoulder blade, moves as we play, automatically and in the appropriate amount. These small movements facilitate and enable the movements of the fingers, hands, and forearms that are usually thought of as constituting technique. When the arms are free, the technique functions better.

To develop a sense of the whole arm, you need to practice moving it. Stand in balance and attend to the feeling of support through your core. Retaining the awareness of support through the core, wave your arms around. As you do this, be sure to include your whole arm in your awareness and in the movement. Feel the collarbone and shoulder blade participate. Trace huge circles with your arms and think of the tip of the scapula as the center of the circle. Swimming movements are good also—most people use their whole arms in swimming. Raise your arm from your side forty-five degrees. Notice that if you continue to raise it higher still, the collarbone and shoulder blade will naturally tend to participate in the movement (provided you do not hold them tense). This is called "humero-scapular rhythm." It feels good, and it is good for you.

Humero-scapular rhythm is a vital concept for pianists. It is vital both as a concept, something to understand, and as a feeling, something to experience (the preceding paragraphs, including the practical "exercises" in italics, are intended to help pianists develop the feeling). The absence of humero-scapular rhythm is a common source of injury. What we spoke of earlier as "fixing" the shoulder blade and collarbone is harmful in part because it inhibits humero-scapular rhythm, which occurs automatically in pianists with good body maps.

THE STERNOCLAVICULAR JOINT

The sternoclavicular joint connects the breastbone (sternum) to the collarbone (clavicle). It is the joint that connects the arm structure to the rest of the skeleton. The sternoclavicular joint permits the collarbone to move in three ways. It can move up and down, forward and back, and it can rotate.

To locate your sternoclavicular joints, place the fingertips of your right hand on your right collarbone and the fingertips of your left hand on your left collarbone. Explore the length of your collarbones with your fingertips, and then let the fingertips move along the length of the collarbone toward the breastbone. When the fingers reach the end of the collarbone, you feel a bony lump and just beyond it is the sternoclavicular joint.

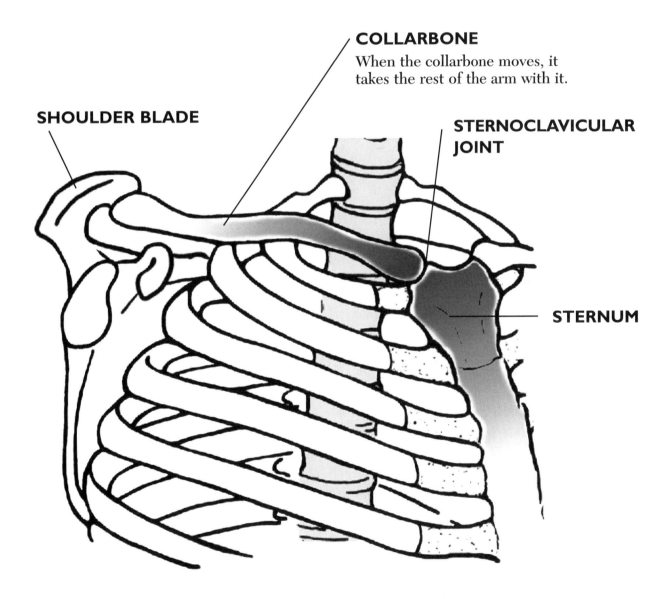

COLLARBONE
When the collarbone moves, it takes the rest of the arm with it.

SHOULDER BLADE

STERNOCLAVICULAR JOINT

STERNUM

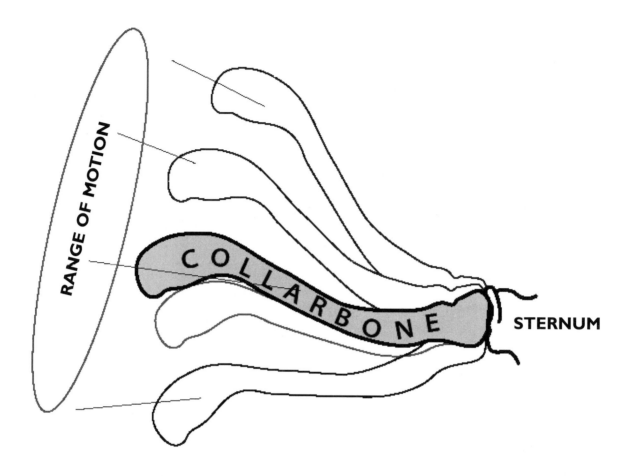

RANGE OF MOTION

COLLARBONE

STERNUM

The collarbone pivots at the sternum.

To appreciate the movement that occurs at the sternoclavicular joint, keep your fingers on the joints and move your collarbones up and down, forward and back. Move them in big circles. Move them as far as you can in all directions while registering with your finger how much motion occurs at the joint. Take a few moments several times a day to explore the range of motion possible for the collarbone. Attend to the way the entire arm moves with the collarbone. Do this regularly until free movement at the sternoclavicular joint has become automatic. People who have been in the habit of keeping the joint fixed may think that not much motion is possible, and when they

first try to move their collarbones, the movements are tiny. Let your collarbone move as far up and down and forward and back as possible. More mobility is available than many people realize.

To become aware of the rotational movement of the collarbone, place the fingers of your left hand at the sternoclavicular joint of the right arm. Hold your right arm bent with your thumb pointing up, in the hitchhiking position, and then turn your entire arm so that the thumb points straight down to the floor. As you do this, your left hand can feel the slight rotation of the collarbone at the sternoclavicular joint.

The rotation of the collarbone at the sterno-clavicular joint is not large, but we need to map it or we will not use it and some pianistic tasks, such as hand crossing or reaching in front of the body, will be more difficult. The collarbone is fixed to the shoulder blade, so the rotation of the collarbone takes the shoulder blade with it. The rotational movement of the collarbone is magnified by the shoulder blade; indeed, some people speak of rotation of the shoulder blade, since that is the more obvious movement, instead of rotation of the collarbone.

Many pianists hold their collarbones and shoulder blades fixed, which means that they inhibit motion at their sternoclavicular joints. Fixing of the sternoclavicular joint inhibits humero-scapular rhythm. One cause of fixing at this joint is the mismapping we call the shoulder-arm split, discussed earlier. If the joint is fixed, there will be too little motion at the sternoclavicular joint and too much at the shoulder joint (leading, sometimes, to rotator cuff injuries and other problems).

We do not normally use large motions at this joint in playing the piano (hand crossing, which is facilitated by a forward movement of the collarbone and shoulder blade, is an exception), but small motions occur constantly if the playing is free. Although the appropriate motions may not be large, they will probably feel large to you at first if you have had a habit of fixing the sternoclavicular joint.

Besides moving too little, most people's collarbones and shoulder blades do not automatically assume an optimal place of rest. The place of rest should be that place from which motion in any direction is easy, the place of equilibrium. In equilibrium the shoulder joints are aligned in the same vertical plane as the other places of balance and the joints face straight out to the sides, like another pair of ears (see the illustration of places of balance, p. 37). All too often, however, the shoulder blades and collarbones do not automatically go to the place of equilibrium. Instead, many people have a habit of pulling the shoulder blades and collarbones down and inwards, that is, they make themselves narrower than their full free width. Others chronically pull their shoulders up and back, or down and back. Any of these habits leaves some muscles chronically stretched, others shortened, and movement of the arms is compromised.

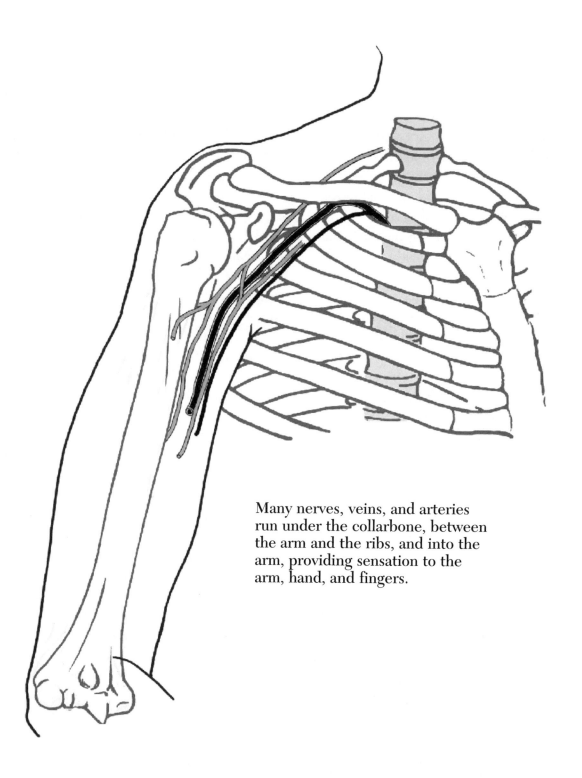

Many nerves, veins, and arteries run under the collarbone, between the arm and the ribs, and into the arm, providing sensation to the arm, hand, and fingers.

If you have numbness in your arms as you play, you are either diseased (see your doctor) or you are putting pressure on these nerves, which is far more common. Ease your neck, release your torso front and back around your core, let your arm structure suspend above these nerves as it should, and your numbness will disappear.

The habit of pulling the shoulder blade and collarbone down is dangerous because if the shoulder blade and collarbone chronically rest too low, the collarbone can put pressure on the nerves that supply the arm. This can produce symptoms of "thoracic outlet syndrome," which resemble those of carpal tunnel syndrome (since the same nerves are affected). The habit of pulling the collarbone and shoulder blade up and back, or down and back, can produce back and shoulder pain.

Lengthening and gathering of the spine must be available in order to have perfect suspension of the arms. Or, putting the point slightly differently, the same muscles that are tensed to pull the collarbone and shoulder blade chronically out of equilibrium also inhibit lengthening and gathering of the spine. This is the basis for my remark in the discussion of lengthening and gathering, where I said, "If you feel that your arms are freely floating, not heavy or constrained in any way, not resting on anything, and you feel that the whole of you is the source of the sound, then you are very likely lengthening and gathering naturally already."

The shoulder blade and collarbone can be taught gradually to balance in a place of equilibrium. The following routine, repeated regularly, will help bring this about.

First, raise your collarbone and shoulder blade up, slowly, as high as you can. Hold them there fore a moment and attend carefully to the muscles you use to do that. Then, very slowly and gradually, release those muscles. Feel them slowly release as the collarbone and shoulder blade descend.

Attending all the time, note the point where the muscles reach a point of feeling "no work." Then stop. It is important that the release be slow and gradual lest, through habit, you go past the point of no work. Although the place you have reached is probably a bit higher than you're used to (assuming that, like many pianists, you've had a habit of pulling the shoulder blade and collarbone down), going lower would actually require the use of other muscles to pull the collarbone and shoulder blade down. Do that next. Pull them down as far as you can and notice the muscles in your back and sides that work when you do that. Feel the muscular work of pulling the collarbone and shoulder blade down. Then very slowly release those muscles. Notice that as you release the muscles your collarbone and shoulder blade rise. Continue until you feel no work in those muscles.

Follow the same steps to move the collarbone and shoulder blade forward as far as possible, then release slowly, allowing them to return to the place of no work. Next, move the collarbone and shoulder blade backward, pulling your shoulder blades together, then release the muscles, slowly returning to the point of no work.

If you do these movements several times a day your shoulder blade and collarbone will gradually learn to rest in the place of equilibrium. It may take time for the new alignment to become habitual, but you can experience its value immediately by trying the following experiment. Play a passage on the piano, then do the above routine and play the passage again. The results are likely to speak for themselves.

ↄ

The movements at the sternoclavicular joint are likely to be somewhat larger for organists than for pianists. For organists who must move from one keyboard to another, free movement at the sternoclavicular joint and the resulting mobility of the shoulder blade and collarbone must be learned and clearly understood. Organists who do not understand this mobility, when required to reach to an upper keyboard, will usually "reach out" with the arms and neck, while at the same time rounding the upper back and rocking back onto the tailbone. This places unwanted tension throughout the back and arm structure, inhibits free playing, and ultimately causes pain.

Free and easy movement at the sternoclavicular joint is also required when both hands are playing in the high range of the keyboards (as in the Widor Toccata V), and when the hands are on separate manuals, especially when the left hand is higher than the right, or the right hand is lower than the left.

ↄ

THE SHOULDER JOINT

The second joint of the arm, the gleno-humeral joint, does have a common name: the shoulder joint. The shoulder joint is not the joint that connects the arm to the body. Thinking of it that way encourages the mismapping called the shoulder-arm split. Nor does the shoulder joint connect the arm to the shoulder, as if the shoulder were a distinct part of the body separate from the arm. The shoulder joint connects two parts of the arm. When the shoulder blade and collarbone move up, down, forward, and back, the shoulder joint also moves. That is, the entire joint moves as part of the arm structure. The shoulder joint is not a fixed place from which the arm moves, it is part of the arm.

The shoulder joint is our most mobile joint. Not only does it permit three kinds of movement—up and down, back and forth, and rotational (the hip joint also permits these three kinds of movement)—it also has a greater range of motion than any other joint. Unfortunately, many pianists hold their shoulder joints fixed and stiff, to the detriment of their playing. Possibly their way of moving is influenced by the common description of the shoulder joint as a "ball and socket." The humerus does end in a ball. If the ball were surrounded by a socket of bone, motion at the shoulder joint would indeed be limited, the way movement of a light bulb in its socket is limited. But that is not the arrangement we have.

SHOULDER BLADE **SHOULDER JOINT** **SHOULDER BLADE**

glenoid fossa of the shoulder blade

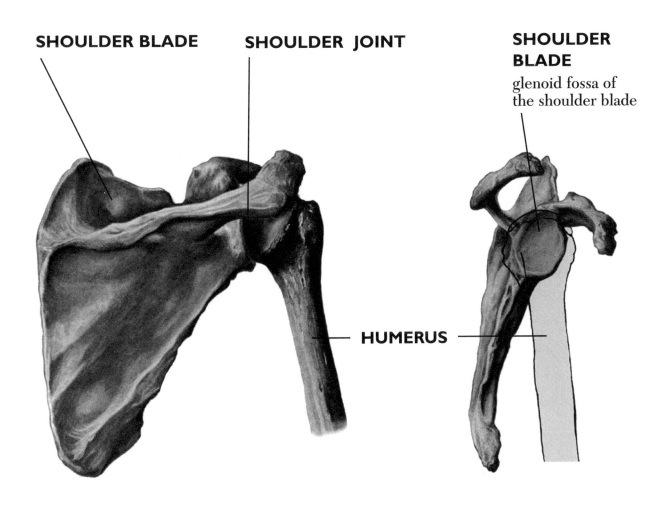

HUMERUS

Shoulder joint
seen from the back.

Shoulder joint
from the side.

The ball at the end of the humerus articulates with a small, basin-shaped surface that forms the outer end of the shoulder blade, the *glenoid fossa* (from which we get the name "glenohumeral joint"). The glenoid fossa is all there is by way of a "socket" for the ball of the humerus. The surface of the glenoid fossa is small, only about the size of a thumb print, and it does not surround the ball of the humerus or constrict its movement. A capsule of ligaments holds the ball of the humerus in position against the fossa; these ligaments are flexible enough to permit an exceptionally wide range of motion. As the humerus moves, the ball turns in different ways and different parts of its surface come in contact with the fossa.

Pianists need to be aware of the shoulder joint, because many pianistic motions require freedom of this joint. Moving the hands to the extremes of the keyboard is an obvious example of movement at the shoulder joint. An example that may not be so obvious is the movement of the hand in and out of the black key area. As a matter of anatomy, when the hand moves into and out of the black key area, movement must occur at the shoulder joint (unless the pianist performs in-and-out movements by moving the entire body forward and back—a poor solution). If the pianist does not map in-and-out movements with awareness that they require freedom at the shoulder joint, the movements may be stiff or may not occur. This happens for some pianists who do not consciously map in-and-out movements at all. It may also happen for some who think of in-and-out motions as initiated from the

forearm, if they forget that the place where they think of "initiation" and the joint where the movement occurs are not the same.

Many pianists hold their shoulder joints tightly and the movements that would make their playing easier do not occur. It helps to think of the shoulder joint being free—move the upper arm back and forth, up and down, experience how mobile the shoulder joint is—and then bring that sensation of freedom to the piano. Suddenly the playing is better because the upper arm movements that permit more perfect hand placement on each note are being allowed to happen. Most people need to spend some time deliberately mapping the movements of the shoulder joint to develop greater freedom.

I have claimed that pianists move too little at the shoulder joint, but, paradoxically, they also move too much. That is, the movement that does occur in the shoulder area is confined to the shoulder joint instead of being appropriately distributed between the shoulder joint and the sternoclavicular joint, as it would be if the arm structure were truly coordinated. The shoulder joint does too much, the sternoclavicular joint too little.

Besides moving up and down, forward and back, the humerus can rotate at the shoulder joint. Pianists need to include this movement in their map of the shoulder joint movements. The pianist who does not map rotation at the shoulder joint may move the upper arm bone toward and away from the body when rotation would be more efficient. Pianists who cultivate one of the techniques based on forearm rotation need to know about rotation at the shoulder joint also, since some motions taught as forearm

---

❧

Free movement at the shoulder joint is necessary for organists, not only to move in and out of the black notes, but to move freely from one keyboard to another.

Sit at the organ and practice moving in and out of the black notes, feeling the movement that occurs at the shoulder joint. Then practice making the same movements moving from one keyboard to another. The movements will be larger, but they are the same movements.

---

rotation are actually rotations at the shoulder joint, not the forearm. For example, a pianist who does not know about rotation at the shoulder joint may have trouble learning the proper rotational technique for ascending scales in the right hand.

Hold your forearm up in front of you and move it back and forth like a windshield wiper. Notice that when you do this, your arm rotates at the shoulder joint. Now bring your forearm parallel to the floor and repeat the rotation as if the windshield wiper were wiping a horizontal windshield. You can see from this that rotation of the shoulder joint is used in piano playing.

There is a rotational release at the shoulder joint that is important for pianists. Many people, when they stand, have their palms facing their legs and their thumbs toward the front of the body. They may tell you, if you ask them, that this is the proper way for the arms to hang. In fact, when the arms hang freely in balance, the palms face backwards. Turning the palms toward the legs requires a rotation of the upper arm away from neutral. The motion occurs at the shoulder joint and is accomplished by

tensing muscles in the upper torso. Releasing that muscular tension allows the shoulder joint to rotate back to neutral and facilitates bringing the hands to the keyboard. If the tension is not released, then there will be tension in the shoulders underlying the playing of every note. The release is analogous to the release of butt muscles that permits the legs to rotate back to neutral, which we discussed earlier in connection with sitting.

Try letting your arms hang at your sides with the palms facing your legs. Bring your hand up to the keyboard with the thumb leading, then pronate the forearm to put the hand into playing position. This movement is sometimes taught as the proper way to bring the hand to the keyboard. The problem with it is that you can do it and still have tension in your shoulder joints. Now let your arms hang at your sides, release any rotational tension in the shoulder joint to permit the palm to face backwards, and bring your hand to the keyboard. Feel that the back of your hand, not your thumb, leads the forearm to the keyboard. It will feel easier, and the hand will be less likely to tilt toward the little finger.

THE ELBOW JOINT

The humerus connects to the forearm at the elbow. The forearm contains two bones: the radius, on the thumb side of the forearm, and the ulna, on the little finger side of the forearm. The elbow joint is thus a joint of one bone with two bones. But only one of the forearm bones, the ulna, actually articulates with the humerus. The radius does not articulate with the humerus. It just sits alongside the ulna and at its end near the elbow it is held in place by a ring-shaped ligament, the anular ligament. Two kinds of motion occur at the elbow joint: bending and rotating.

Bending: The bending and unbending of the elbow joint occur at the joint of the ulna with the humerus. Instead of smooth articular surfaces that would permit motion of several kinds (as at the shoulder joint), the ulna and humerus have grooves and ridges that fit into each other and prevent every kind of motion except bending and its opposite, unbending. Where few kinds of motion are possible, few muscles are needed. Just three principal muscles are involved in bending and unbending at the elbow joint: the biceps and brachialis to bend, the triceps to unbend. This is in contrast to the large number of muscles that move the arm in myriad ways at the shoulder joint.

Rotation: The other important movement of the forearm is rotation. Rotation of the forearm permits the palm of the hand to face up (supination) or down (pronation). Free rotation of the forearm permits movement of about 180 degrees from fully supinated to fully pronated. Rotation is independent of bending and unbending. You can bend and unbend your elbow with your palm facing up or with your palm facing down, or anything in between.

Forearm rotation is constantly used in piano playing. Some very efficient pianists deliberately practice rotation, using tiny rotations of the forearm in conjunction with finger movements. But even pianists who do not consciously train forearm rotation as an element of technique still use it, since the mere bringing of the hands into playing position with the palms facing the floor requires pronation of the forearm. Therefore all pianists, whether they are aware of it or not, rotate their forearms to play the piano.

The proper mapping of forearm rotation is absolutely vital for pianists. If forearm rotation is mismapped and a person rotates in a way that involves chronic tension, the result is disaster. Improper mapping of forearm rotation is a major source of limitation, pain, and injury among pianists (and other musicians, too, as well as computer users, writers, and others). Many, perhaps most, cases of pain and tendonitis in the forearm are caused by mismapping forearm rotation, and are cured when the map is corrected. Every pianist needs to grasp the mechanics of forearm rotation with perfect clarity and use that understanding to cultivate kinesthetic awareness. For many injured pianists, this is the most important part of the book.

When the palm faces up (supination), the two bones in the forearm are parallel. When the palm faces down, as in playing the piano (pronation), they are crossed. But although the bones are parallel in one case, crossed in the other, only one of them actually moves. Take a moment to feel your forearm while you rotate it, and try to ascertain which bone moves and which one is stationary.

THE ELBOW JOINT (RIGHT ARM, PALM UP)

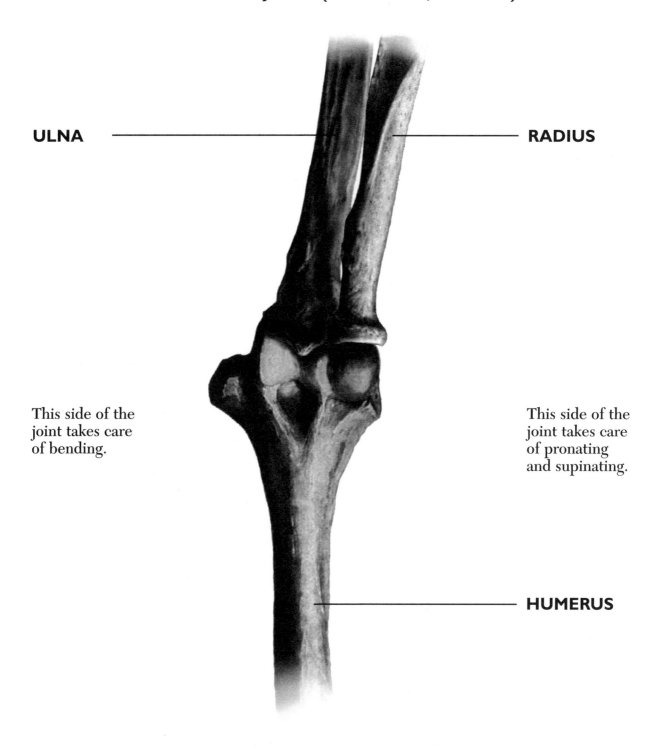

ULNA

RADIUS

This side of the joint takes care of bending.

This side of the joint takes care of pronating and supinating.

HUMERUS

Hold your right hand out in front of you, palm up, and look at your elbow. If you could see the bones of your elbow joint, this is what you would see.

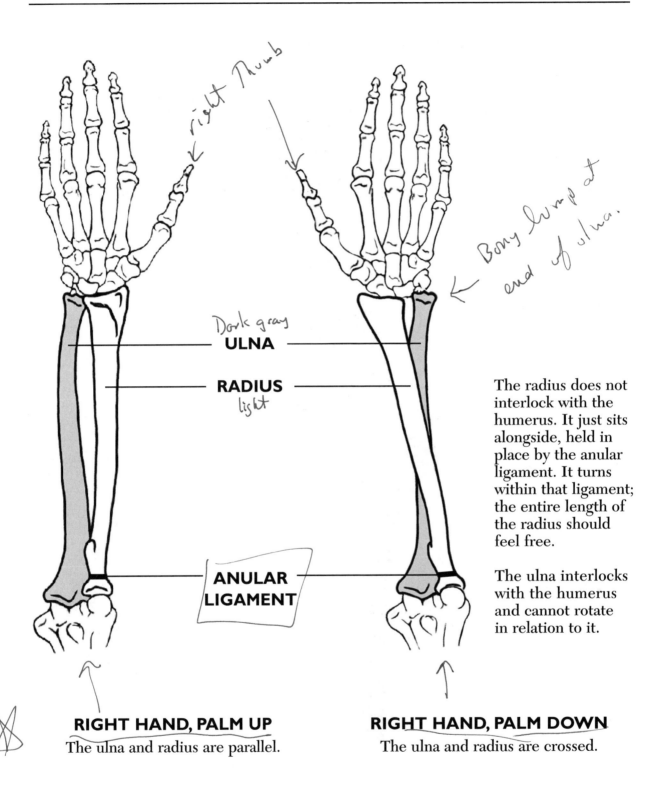

right Thumb

Bony lump at end of ulna.

Dark gray
ULNA

RADIUS
light

ANULAR LIGAMENT

The radius does not interlock with the humerus. It just sits alongside, held in place by the anular ligament. It turns within that ligament; the entire length of the radius should feel free.

The ulna interlocks with the humerus and cannot rotate in relation to it.

RIGHT HAND, PALM UP
The ulna and radius are parallel.

RIGHT HAND, PALM DOWN
The ulna and radius are crossed.

If you discovered that the ulna remains stationary when the forearm rotates, congratulations! The radius is the bone that moves. You can verify this as follows: look at the bony lump above your wrist, behind your

fifth finger. That is the end of the ulna. Starting there, you can walk the fingers of the other hand along the ulna to the elbow (you can feel the ulna, just below the skin, along its entire length). Spread your fingertips along the ulna and, while holding them there, rotate your forearm. You will feel that the ulna remains stationary while the forearm rotates. Knowing which forearm bone rotates and which is stationary can make the difference between free, expressive playing and injury. *Right way to rotate*

Rotate your forearm while thinking of the little finger side of the arm as the axis of rotation. You can imagine a line extending along the side of your forearm and including your little finger, then rotate your forearm around that axis. This is "little finger orientation." It feels easy and free because it is in accordance with your structure. An image that helps many people is this: think of your hand as a book, with the ulna and little finger as the spine of the book and the thumb as one of the turning pages; rotate your entire forearm to turn the page.

Now contrast the feeling of little finger orientation with what happens if you think of the other side of your arm as the axis. Imagine a line up the other side of the forearm and including the thumb. Rotate your forearm around that imaginary axis. This is "thumb orientation." Thumb orientation is the result of mismapping the radius as the stationary bone. It feels stiff and awkward compared to little finger orientation. Notice that when you become thumb oriented the entire hand tends to turn toward the little finger—it twists, that is, toward the ulna, in what is called "ulnar deviation." Chronic ulnar deviation is a characteristic symptom of thumb-oriented movement.

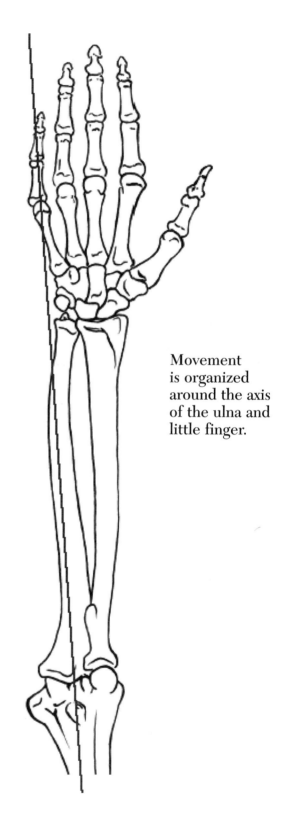

Movement is organized around the axis of the ulna and little finger.

Little finger orientation.
Right arm, palm up.

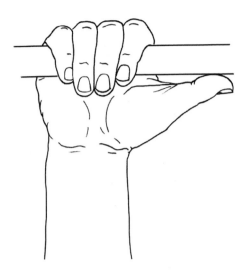

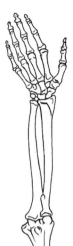

Right arm, palm up.

Suspension from a bar with little finger orientation is strong and secure.

Here is a way to develop awareness of the organization of movement in the arms. Place your right hand, palm down, on top of your left hand, with the tips of the fingers of your left hand touching the outside of the little finger of your right hand. Then raise your right hand above your head and as you do so allow the fingers of your left hand to slide along your right arm, along the ulna and the humerus and all the way to the tip of your shoulder blade. Trace the same path on your left hand and arm, using your right hand. Feel the line you have traced as organizing the relationships and movements of the entire arms and hands. What you have traced is the organization of the arm as it exists for all creatures capable of hanging from a branch or a bar. The same organization that carries a creature from branch to branch in the forest carries our arms over the keyboard. Be aware of little finger orientation of your hand and forearm and put it into the perspective of the entire arm. Notice the feeling of freedom in the thumb that

Thumb orientation usually leads to chronic ulnar deviation.

becomes available when movement is little-finger oriented. Bring this organization to the piano and keep it in your awareness, never losing it for even an instant, as you slowly try different pianistic tasks. If you have a habit of thumb orientation you may need to alter your technique to retain the sense of little finger orientation

A helpful way of thinking is this: in thumb-oriented ulnar deviation, movement is *directed toward* the little finger (bad). In little finger orientation, movement is *organized around* the little finger (good).

The hand is connected to the radius by the wrist. At the wrist joint, the shapes of the articulating surfaces of the radius and the wrist bones determine the sorts of motion that are possible. The hand can move up and down (as in waving) and it can bend sideways in each direction. But the hand cannot rotate in relation to the radius, as many musicians imagine it to do. Serious injury can result from imagining that pronation and supination of the hand occur at the wrist. The hand rotates with the radius, around the ulna. Thinking of the hand and radius as rotating together helps to keep the rotation as free as possible.

The sideways movement of the hand toward the little finger is called ulnar deviation because the hand bends toward the ulna; sideways movement of the hand toward the thumb is called radial deviation because the hand bends toward the radius. That we can move our hands sideways this way is an important fact about us; special features of our structure make it possible. If you palpate the place just in front of the bony lump at the end of the ulna, with the hand held straight, you can feel a space between the ulna and the wrist bones. This space permits ulnar deviation. If you allow the hand to deviate toward the little finger you will feel the space close. Other primates cannot do this. Our human structure permits it and

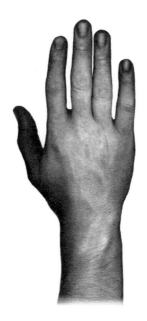

Little finger orientation permits free movement without tension.

BAD

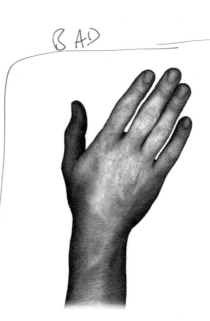

Ulnar deviation looks like this and is usually a sign of thumb orientation.

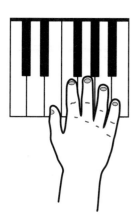 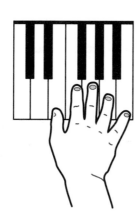

The hand should look like the one on the left, with a long, easy wrist, not like the one on the right, with the wrist tight and strained.

thus permits movements that are vital for certain activities and may well have contributed to the development of human intelligence. In particular, this movement helps make it possible to hold a stick and use it as a tool or club. Grip a stick or pencil and hold it so that it points directly forward, making an extension of the arm. This way of grasping extends our repertoire of movements. But look at your hand when you do it and you'll see that the hand is turned toward the ulna. It is "ulnar deviating."

Chronic ulnar deviation is a principal cause of stress injury. And yet the ability to do it is an important feature of the human hand. How does it come about that such an important movement can be dangerous?

The answer is this: the position of the hand is not what is dangerous, it is the quality of movement used to assume the position that may or may not be dangerous. If a person assumes an ulnar-deviated position of the hand using thumb-oriented movements, which is what many pianists do, then the person is at risk. But when forearm rotation is properly mapped, the hand can deviate without thumb orientation. In that case ulnar deviation is benign. There are pianists who deviate in both directions without injury. If a person deviates freely, oriented around the ulna, then the amount of deviation to use is a choice the person can make. Some pianists use a lot, some scarcely any.

However, having said that the mere position of ulnar deviation is not what is dangerous, but rather the thumb-oriented way of assuming the position, I must add that few pianists who use a lot of ulnar deviation do so safely. Usually, the position of ulnar deviation

is a symptom of thumb-oriented movement. That is why some people have concluded that the position itself is what is dangerous. But the position is just a clue, it does not give the whole story. Sometimes a person can be thumb oriented even though the position of the hand is not deviated very much. In such a case, the outward appearance of the hand will seem acceptable but will be misleading. What matters is the quality of movement underlying the position.

Organists, read and study this section on forearm rotation several times! The most common and debilitating injuries organists suffer are the result of mismapping forearm rotation. Thumb-oriented movements are always risky, but when combined with the movements involved in changing manuals, such improper movements can be devastating.

THE THREE ROTATIONS OF THE ARM: SUMMARY

There are three rotational movements of the arm. All three rotations are used in piano playing and should be part of a pianist's body map.

1. Rotation of the collarbone and shoulder blade at the sternoclavicular joint, as when we cross our hands or reach across the front of the body to the extremes of the keyboard.

1. The rotation of the shoulder blade over the ribs moves the whole arm structure forward or back at the sternoclavicular joint.

2. The rotation at the shoulder joint turns the arm without changing the bend or rotation at the elbow.

3. The rotation at the elbow turns the hand over.

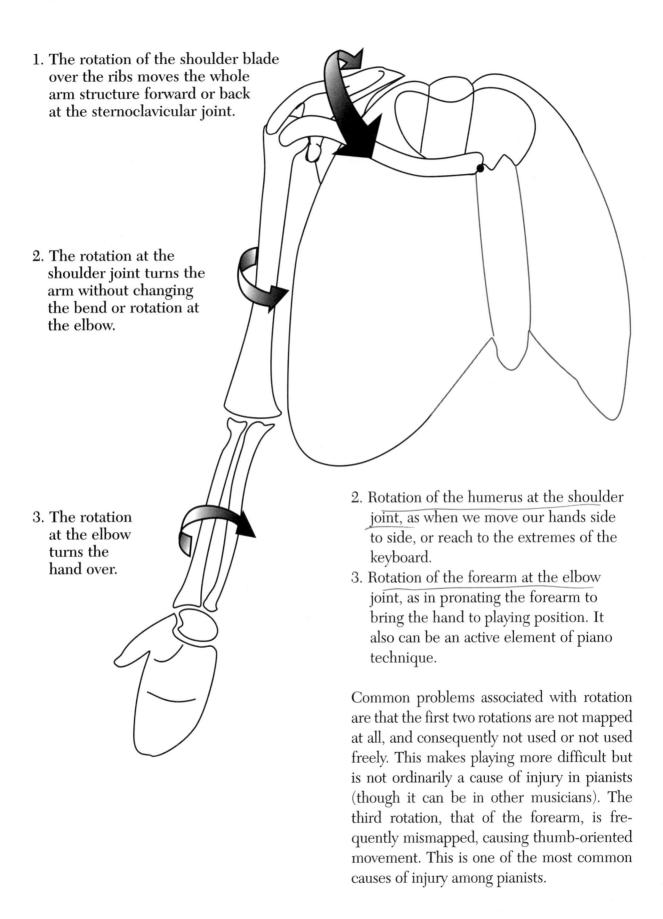

2. Rotation of the humerus at the shoulder joint, as when we move our hands side to side, or reach to the extremes of the keyboard.
3. Rotation of the forearm at the elbow joint, as in pronating the forearm to bring the hand to playing position. It also can be an active element of piano technique.

Common problems associated with rotation are that the first two rotations are not mapped at all, and consequently not used or not used freely. This makes playing more difficult but is not ordinarily a cause of injury in pianists (though it can be in other musicians). The third rotation, that of the forearm, is frequently mismapped, causing thumb-oriented movement. This is one of the most common causes of injury among pianists.

THE WRIST

We saw earlier that the knee is a joint, not a structure. The wrist, by contrast, is both a joint and a structure. As a structure, it lies between the forearm and the hand. It is composed of eight bones, called carpal bones. The carpals are arranged in two rows of four.

To locate your wrist, look at the back of your right hand, then at the bony lump on the right side of your forearm, six or eight inches from your little fingertip. That is the end of the ulna, and it marks the end of your forearm. The wrist is in front of that lump, closer to your hand. The wrist occupies about two inches between the end of the ulna and the hand. If you look at your palm, the wrist structure extends about one inch

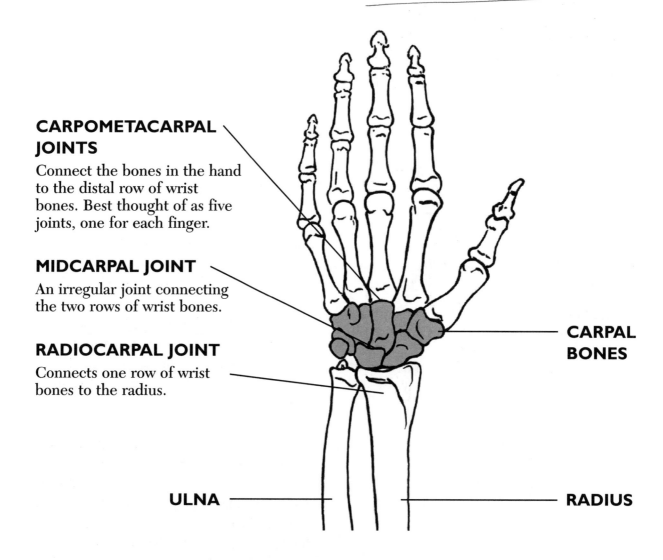

CARPOMETACARPAL JOINTS

Connect the bones in the hand to the distal row of wrist bones. Best thought of as five joints, one for each finger.

MIDCARPAL JOINT

An irregular joint connecting the two rows of wrist bones.

RADIOCARPAL JOINT

Connects one row of wrist bones to the radius.

CARPAL BONES

ULNA

RADIUS

The wrist is a flexible structure, two rows of small bones connecting the arm and hand.
Right arm, palm up.

into the fleshy part of your hand; the beginning of your palm does not indicate the end of the wrist. The appearance of the palm side of the hand does not reflect the underlying structure of the wrist (the same is true of the knuckles, as we shall see). Pianists who map the hand from the palm side develop problems.

The wrist is not the narrowest part of your arm. The narrowest part, for most people, is behind the lump that marks the end of the ulna. If you wear your watch, as many people do, on the narrow part of your arm behind the lump of your ulna, your watch is on your forearm, not on your wrist.

Besides being a structure about two inches long, the wrist is a joint, one of the four major joints of the arm. Pianists should think of it, however, not as one joint but a series of three joints. The first joint connects the forearm to the first row of wrist bones, the second connects the first row to the second row of wrist bones, and the third connects the second row of wrist bones to the hand.

Since the forearm contains two bones, the joint connecting the forearm to the first row of wrist bones might be a joint of two bones with four. But that is not really the situation. The wrist bones articulate with just one bone of the forearm, the radius. The ulna does not articulate with the wrist bones, it just sits alongside, much as the radius sits alongside at the elbow joint. Because the first joint connects the radius to the first row of carpal bones, it is called the radiocarpal joint. At the radiocarpal joint, the radius has a concave elliptical surface. The first row of wrist bones combine to form a corresponding convex elliptical surface. This shape permits two kinds of motion: up-and-down movements of the hand (flexion and extension) and sideways bending (radial and ulnar deviation). It does not permit rotational movements of the wrist and hand in relation to the radius. The hand rotates with the radius, not apart from it. Trying to rotate the hand at the wrist always results in strain and often in inflammation of the wrist. The joint between the two rows of wrist bones (carpals) is the midcarpal joint, and the joint between the second row of carpals and the hand is called the carpometacarpal joint (because it connects the carpal bones to the bones of the hand, the metacarpals).

Because the wrist joint is really a series of three joints, it is not a simple hinge. And because the wrist is a structure with joints in it, it is a flexible structure. The greatest range of wrist movement occurs at the radiocarpal joint, but significant movement occurs at the other joints as well.

Pianists should think of their wrists as long and flexible. In very free movement at the wrist there is an impression, visually and kinesthetically, of lengthening across the wrist in movement. This is distinctly unlike the compression we see in the movement of some pianists in which the wrist actually appears to shorten, the result of an uncomfortable tightening, as if the person were trying to compress the flexible structure into a single hinge. Pianists who think of the wrist as a hinge should immediately correct their maps.

You can experience "lengthening across the wrist" this way: holding your forearm slightly out to the side, move your hand up and down in a waving motion. Try to concentrate all the movement exactly at the end of the forearm and nowhere else. That is the "hinge" movement. Notice the way your hand looks when you do that. Next, release your wrist and move your hand up and down with the sense that your wrist is long and flexible, like a snake. You should find that this way of moving looks and feels very different from the "hinge" movement.

Mapping the wrist joints accurately produces greater freedom of movement. Pianists who cultivate mobility of these joints will develop flexible, supple wrists and hands. This, along with little finger orientation, keeps wrists safe from injury.

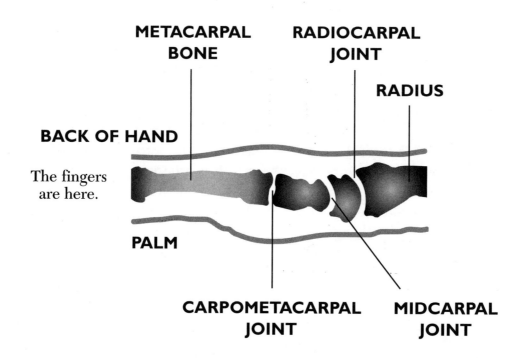

Bones of the wrist seen from the side.

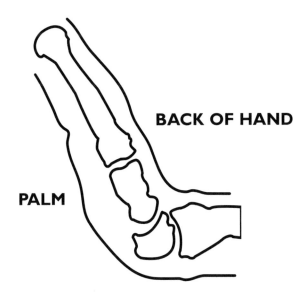

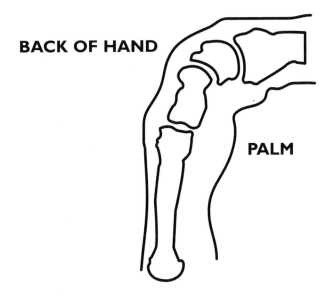

In bending the wrist, most of the movement occurs
at the radiocarpal joint, but significant movement
occurs at the other joints also.

THE HAND

The hand is made up of nineteen bones. There are five metacarpals connected to the bones of the wrist, and fourteen phalanges (two for the thumb and three for each of the other fingers) connected to the metacarpals.

On a skeleton the fingers appear to be very long and they attach directly to the bones of the wrist. The reason the fingers look longer on a skeleton than on a living hand is that on a living hand the metacarpals have muscles between them and ligaments connecting them and are covered over with skin, which makes the hand look like a wide, flat structure with fingers growing out of it. As a result, instead of thinking of a wrist with fingers attached to it we think of a wrist with a hand attached to it and fingers attached to the hand. Almost everyone maps the hand on the basis of that image. If you ask people where the fingers start they will point to the joint of the fingers with the hand, not the joint of the hand with the wrist.

But pianists should map their hands on the basis of the underlying structure, not the appearance. We should feel that our fingers do not end at the knuckles, they end only at the carpometacarpal joint—where they connect with the wrist bones—and they include the metacarpal bones.

We can summarize the discussion of the hand and wrist up to this point by contrasting good and bad maps of the wrist and hand.

Bad map: a forearm connected by a hinge to a hand, and hand connected at the knuckles to the fingers.

Good map: the radius connected to a flexible wrist (three joints), which connects to the fingers.

Note that the good map does not include a hand—or, better, it does not include a hand distinct from the fingers. Note also that in the good map it is the radius, not just "the forearm," that connects to the wrist.

The bones of the hand are connected by nineteen joints (including the carpometacarpal joints that connect the hand to the wrist). Unfortunately, these joints do not have unambiguous common names in English, so we must use technical names or risk misunderstanding. The technical names are cumbersome, so I shall use abbreviations: for example, "MCP joint of the index finger" to refer to the MetaCarpoPhalangeal joint of the index finger, or "DIP joint of the fifth finger" to refer to the Distal InterPhalangeal joint of the fifth finger (see the illustration opposite).

Using the technical names of the bones and joints of the hand is admittedly a bit of a nuisance. I apologize to my readers for that, but I have not discovered any other way to avoid ambiguity and confusion. I urge readers to think of it this way: learning the technical names and abbreviations is far less challenging intellectually than learning the Minuet in G from the Anna Magdalena Bach notebook, which is accomplished with ease by many seven-year-old children.

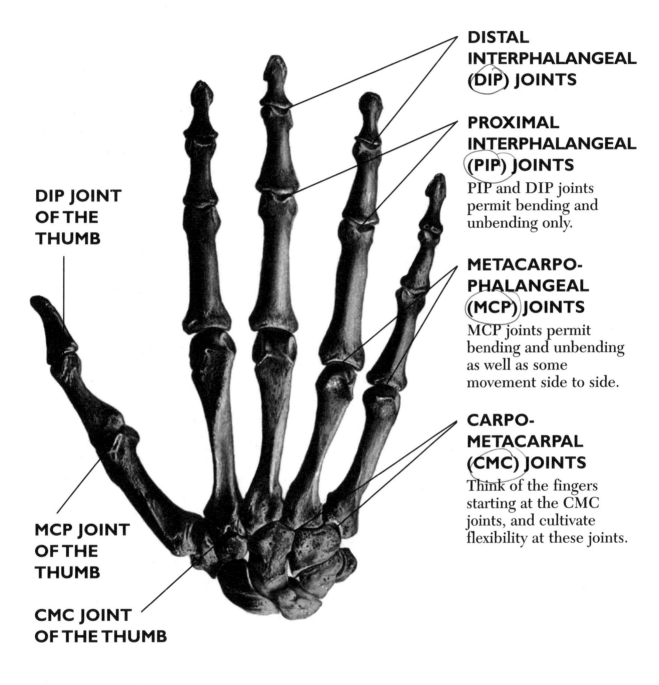

DISTAL INTERPHALANGEAL (DIP) JOINTS

PROXIMAL INTERPHALANGEAL (PIP) JOINTS

PIP and DIP joints permit bending and unbending only.

METACARPO-PHALANGEAL (MCP) JOINTS

MCP joints permit bending and unbending as well as some movement side to side.

CARPO-METACARPAL (CMC) JOINTS

Think of the fingers starting at the CMC joints, and cultivate flexibility at these joints.

DIP JOINT OF THE THUMB

MCP JOINT OF THE THUMB

CMC JOINT OF THE THUMB

Joints of the hand and fingers.

I stressed above that pianists cannot afford to regard the wrist joint as a single joint but must map it as three joints. When we turn to the fingers we find that the third wrist joint, the CMC joint, which connects the wrist to the fingers, is really a complex joint and cannot be regarded as a single joint by pianists. The fingers move separately at this joint, in different amounts. Motion of the three middle fingers is small but perceptible; motion of the fifth finger is fairly large, and motion of the thumb is very large—in fact, the CMC joint is the principal joint for motion of the thumb. Therefore, pianists should regard the CMC joint as five joints, one for each finger.

Using one hand to massage the other, locate the CMC joints. Explore the range of motion possible for each finger at this joint. Do this regularly to develop as much flexibility in the hand as you can.

Developing maximum freedom of the CMC joints facilitates playing chords and octaves. Although the amount of motion at the CMC joints may seem small, any additional freedom you achieve here will be magnified at the tips of your fingers. Cultivate the feeling that the entire hand encompasses the chord or octave. You should not think of merely spreading your fingers but use the entire hand. Chances are that if you have been accustomed to thinking of "stretching" or "spreading" your fingers, replacing that thought with the idea of using your entire hand will by itself produce greater ease in chords and octaves.

Another point in connection with chords and octaves is that you should not "set" your hand before playing the chord or octave, nor in a series of octaves should you keep your hand fixed in position as you move from one to the next. Setting the hand in advance, or holding it fixed in position, simply creates tension. You can allow your hand to fall on the chord or octave without setting it in advance, and you'll play with less tension. Trust it, you won't miss (or you'll learn not to). Chords and octaves will feel effortless in comparison to how they feel with the hand fixed in position. An image that helps many pianists open the hand by just the right amount is "let the piano open your hand." Be sure to think of the opening of your hand not as a spreading of the fingers but as an opening from the CMC joints, like an umbrella. Some pianists who learn to use the whole hand and eliminate the tension involved in fixing the hand can actually extend their reach.

USE OF THE THUMB

Belief that the finger starts at the MCP joint is especially harmful in the case of the thumb. Many people, if you ask them where their thumb starts, point to the MCP joint, not to the CMC joint where the thumb connects to the bones of the wrist. They will say that the thumb has only two bones, and they will try to move the thumb from the MCP joint. Quite often, the MCP joint of the thumb will be quite prominent in these people, an indication that they have not mapped their thumbs properly. They can sometimes exhibit considerable mobility at that joint. But mobility of the MCP joint is usually a compensation for loss of movement at the CMC joint. The muscles surrounding the metacarpal bone of the thumb will be tense and hard. Often the tension extends to the entire forearm as well.

This mismapping of the thumb, and the tension that results from it, is a frequent cause of

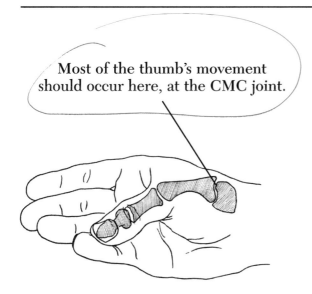

Most of the thumb's movement should occur here, at the CMC joint.

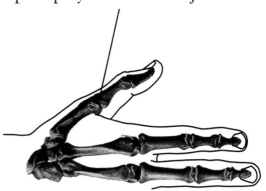

The thumb should not move principally from the MCP joint.

If you are using your whole thumb, one that includes three joints, you will feel a secure and comfortable relationship with the instrument. If you are assuming that the thumb is two bones instead of three, you will suffer from restricted movement at the CMC joint, nearest the wrist, an over-prominence at the MCP joint, and probably soreness as well.

injury. Therefore, pianists who think of the thumb as consisting of just two bones and try to move it that way should immediately undertake to correct their maps and habituate themselves to the free movement of the thumb, all three bones of it, from the CMC joint. The articular surfaces of the bones at the CMC joint of the thumb are saddle-shaped, permitting a wide range of up-and-down motion and sideways motion (but not rotation). Restoring full freedom and mobility to that joint, if it has been fixed, may take some weeks and will require a deliberate focusing of attention. It is essential for greater ease in playing and for injury prevention.

If the CMC joint of your thumb does not move easily, or if you tend to move the thumb more at the MCP joint than at the CMC joint, you should undertake to restore mobility at the CMC joint. Massage the area around the metacarpal bone of the thumb and allow the muscles to release as much as possible. Move that bone back and forth, encouraging mobility at the CMC joint. Be aware that all three bones of the thumb move as one. Practice passing the thumb across the palm to touch the tips of the various fingers, being sure that the thumb moves from the CMC joint. Notice that when the thumb touches the fifth finger (as in the illustration on the left on this page), the fifth finger also moves from its own CMC joint. Do this frequently until proper movement of the thumb is automatic.

The movement of the thumb to touch the little finger, with both the thumb and little finger moving at their CMC joints, illustrates the "opposable thumb" that separates our hands from the hands (or paws) of almost all other creatures, and makes our hands capable of performing a bewildering variety of tasks. This is also the movement used to pass the thumb, or cross over the thumb, in piano playing. Passing the thumb under should be a movement of the thumb at the CMC joint, not at the MCP joint. Also, in passing the thumb, the thumb should move only as far as it can go without tension; it should not be fixed or squeezed under the hand.

Some pianists believe that whereas fingers 2–5 play on the ends of the fingers, the thumb plays on its side, contacting the key with the side of the distal phalanx. In fact, there are many pianistic situations where the most efficient point of contact with the key is the "front corner" of the thumb, not the side. This is often true in arpeggios, or situations of going from a black key played with a long finger to a white key played with the thumb. In such situations, playing too far down on the side of the thumb puts the entire arm lower and hampers movement to whatever note comes after the thumb. In other situations, such as playing white key trills using 1 and 3, it is indeed easier to use the side of the thumb.

Experiment with different points of contact for the thumb. Using the front corner of the thumb facilitates some passages enormously. Notice, though, that if you have been playing the thumb on its side, using the front corner instead of the side may put your entire forearm at a higher level than you've been accustomed to. That realignment of the forearm can be helpful, but for it to work properly the shoulder joint and sterno-clavicular joint must also be free to move.

Although the thumb moves principally from the CMC joint, it does not move in isolation from the rest of the arm when we play the piano. When the thumb is efficiently used it receives support from the entire forearm through the forearm "arch." There can be a very slight feeling of tilting or rotation in the forearm in the playing of the thumb to distribute the effort across the entire forearm, giving a sense of stability with virtually no effort. Knowledge of the mechanics of forearm rotation ensures that the slight rotational support for the thumb does not lead to thumb orientation. The thumb can remain very free, with the muscles around it loose.

⟶

MOVEMENT OF THE FINGERS AT THE MCP JOINTS

As we have seen, the thumb moves principally from the CMC joint. The other fingers also move at their CMC joints, but the movements are small. The largest movements for fingers 2–5 occur at the MCP joint, sometimes called the "main knuckle." It is vital for pianists to understand what movements the MCP joint permits and what movements it does not permit. Many pianists have been injured by exercises undertaken in the name of stretching the fingers. The injury comes about because what they understand by stretching the fingers is a movement that is inherently tense and potentially injurious. When we understand what movements are possible at the MCP joint, we can avoid those injures.

First, every pianist should locate the MCP joints. That is easy to do. When you look at the back of your hand, the joint is obvious. It is the "main knuckle," the place where people who don't know that the fingers extend back to the wrist would say that the finger joins the hand. Notice, however, that although the joint is obvious on the back of the hand, it is not so obvious on the palm side of the hand. The crease that appears to separate the fingers from the palm does not coincide with the joint. It is in front of the actual joint. If someone imagines that the crease between the palm and the fingers indicates the location of the joint, movement will be stiff. Moreover, mapping the joint that way causes the back of the hand to narrow and arch upward. Therefore, be careful to think of the actual joint, not the crease

between the palm and the fingers, as the place of movement.

The fingers move at the MCP joint in two ways: up and down (flexion and extension), and sideways (abduction and adduction).

Up-and-down movements of the fingers at the MCP joints are free and easy. They are used constantly in playing the piano and are the finger movements that are most obvious to observers. However, it is a bad idea to try to

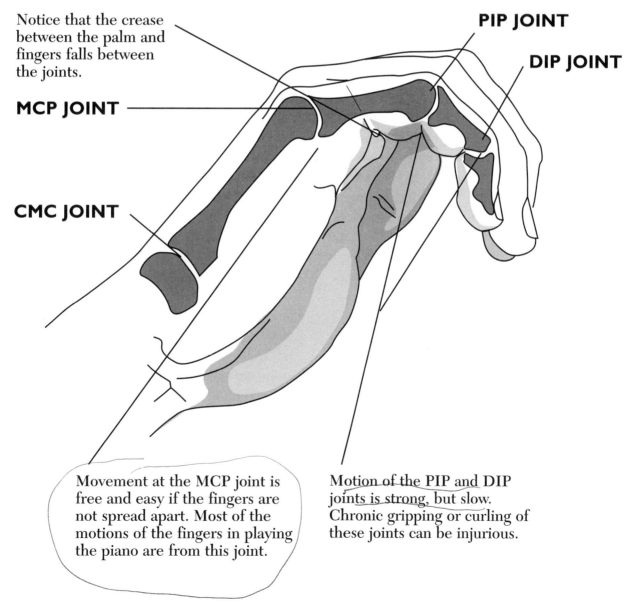

Notice that the crease between the palm and fingers falls between the joints.

PIP JOINT

DIP JOINT

MCP JOINT

CMC JOINT

Movement at the MCP joint is free and easy if the fingers are not spread apart. Most of the motions of the fingers in playing the piano are from this joint.

Motion of the PIP and DIP joints is strong, but slow. Chronic gripping or curling of these joints can be injurious.

move only at the MCP joint. Concentrating movement in the MCP joint alone isolates the fingers from the remainder of the arm and creates tension. Pianists need to be aware of the fingers extending back from the MCP joint to the wrist (the CMC joint) and they need to be aware of the finger as part of a whole arm.

Sideways movements at the MCP joint are called abduction (moving apart) and adduction (moving together). You can experience this movement by holding up fingers 2 and 3 to make a V sign. You can open the V (abduction) or close it (adduction). Notice that abduction and adduction at the MCP joint is slower and more difficult than up-and-down movements. I shall refer to abducting at the MCP joint as stretching or spreading the fingers.

We saw in discussing the elbow joint that bending at the elbow and rotating the forearm are independent of one another; we can rotate our forearms with our elbows bent or straight or anywhere in between. The movements of flexing and abducting the fingers at the MCP joint are not independent in that sense. Try the following movements:

1. *Move fingers 2–5, all together, up and down as freely as you can, at the MCP joint. Notice that as you bend (flex) the MCP joint, the tips of your fingers tend to move closer together.*
2. *Make a V with fingers 2 and 3. Now bend fingers 2 and 3 at the MCP joint. Notice that the V closes—the tips of your fingers come together—the further you bend at the MCP joint.*
3. *Now bend fingers 2–5 simultaneously at the MCP joint. With the fingers bent that way, try to spread them apart. They will not spread at all.*

(Any slight motion you achieve is the result of the MCP joints themselves moving farther apart from each other because of motion at the CMC joints.)

What you have just experienced is grounded in two vital facts that pianists need to understand. First, the curvature of the carpal bones at the CMC joints causes the metacarpal bones and the phalanges to move in planes that are oblique to one another, not parallel. This is the reason for #1 and #2 above.

Second, we cannot simultaneously spread (abduct) the fingers and bend at the MCP joint. This is the reason for #3 above. Abducting the fingers at the MCP joint is possible only when the joint is extended (straight), not when it is flexed (bent). The reason is that there is a ligament, the collateral ligament, on each side of the MCP joint. This ligament is slack when the joint is straight and taut when the joint is bent. When the joint is bent and the ligament is taut it prevents the finger from adducting or abducting. It also makes up-and-down movements more difficult with the fingers spread apart. No amount of practicing will change this anatomical fact, nor will any amount of manually pushing the fingers apart change the fact that they will not abduct when the MCP joint is bent. Many of the exercises aimed at stretching the fingers merely encourage pianists to work against their own anatomy, sometimes to the point of injury.

Moving the fingers up and down while holding them spread apart, in arpeggios, for example, cannot be (i.e., it is anatomically impossible for it to be) as fast and easy as motions with the fingers close together. It generates tension and courts injury. An efficient, safe technique will not attempt to move the fingers rapidly up and down while holding them spread apart, nor will it use spreading or stretching the fingers as a means of covering distances in single-note playing. Instead it will train the arm to move sideways to cover the distances while keeping the fingers in the neutral position from which they can move freely.

As a further exploration of the facts just presented, experiment with playing arpeggios. Try the arpeggio first with the fingers spread over the notes of the chord and remaining over the notes they have already played. Then play the arpeggio without spreading the fingers, neither reaching ahead to anticipate the next note nor lingering over a note already played. This requires sideways movements of the arm—what some teachers describe as letting the arm be "behind" each playing finger.

Moving this way will take some getting used to if you have been playing with your fingers spread apart, but once learned it permits much greater ease and speed, and helps to avoid injury.

ॐ

PHALANGEAL JOINTS

The second and third joints of the fingers, the PIP joints and DIP joints, move only by bending and unbending, which I shall also call "curling" and "uncurling." Movements at the PIP and DIP joints can be used in piano playing, depending on one's technique, but pianists do need to be aware of the dangers of habitually curling these joints without proper release. Notice that though the curling movements are very strong they are not very fast or easy compared to the up-and-down movements at the MCP joint. The reasons for this will emerge in the chapter on muscles.

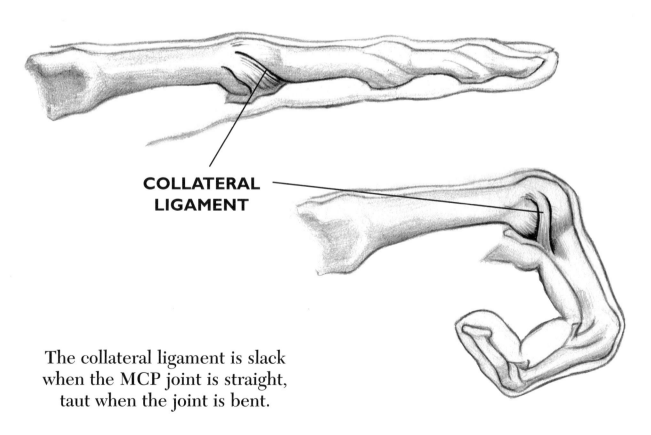

COLLATERAL LIGAMENT

The collateral ligament is slack when the MCP joint is straight, taut when the joint is bent.

CHAPTER 5: MAPPING MUSCLES

Our body map includes the structure, size, and function of the different parts of the body. "Structure" as we have discussed it so far means the bony structure—in most activities we don't need to think about our muscles to move freely. But the body map that suffices for ordinary activities is not adequate for pianists. Pianists need to know about the muscles that move the arms and fingers in order to understand why proper organization of movement makes such a difference. Knowing the roles of the different layers of back muscles is also supremely important for pianists.

When we move our arms or legs, or parts of them, the basic scheme of movement is this: two bones connect to each other at a joint that permits movement, a muscle attaches to one of the bones, crosses the joint, and attaches to the other bone. When the muscle contracts, it pulls on the bones and they move, bending the joint between them. Muscles exert force only when they contract, therefore each muscle can produce movement in only one direction. A different muscle, the *opposing muscle*, is required to produce movement in the opposite direction.

When we move, our kinesthetic sense informs us of our movement and position. Most of the receptors of our kinesthetic sense are in the joints and connective tissue; only a few are in the body of the muscles.

Therefore, although we are aware of movement and position we usually are not aware of the chain of causes, including the neurons and muscles, that bring about the movement.

As an example of the way our kinesthetic sense informs us of movement but not the cause of movement, try curling and uncurling your fingers. You can feel the fingers curling and uncurling. As you do this your awareness of your fingers probably is more vivid than your awareness of your forearm. In fact, you may be aware only of the fingers, not the forearm at all. Nevertheless, the muscles that curl and uncurl your fingers are in the forearm, not in the fingers.

～

THE BACK

The first picture on page 102 shows the deepest layer of back muscles. These muscles attach to adjacent or nearby vertebrae and to the ribs. The second picture shows the next layer of back muscles, which attach to vertebrae distant from each other as well as to ribs and pelvis. These two layers of muscles are "postural" muscles. They work to bend and unbend the spine, make it twist and spiral, and they keep it from bending too far. They make constant adjustments to keep us balanced as we walk, sit, and go about our activities. Their action is mostly automatic or reflexive.

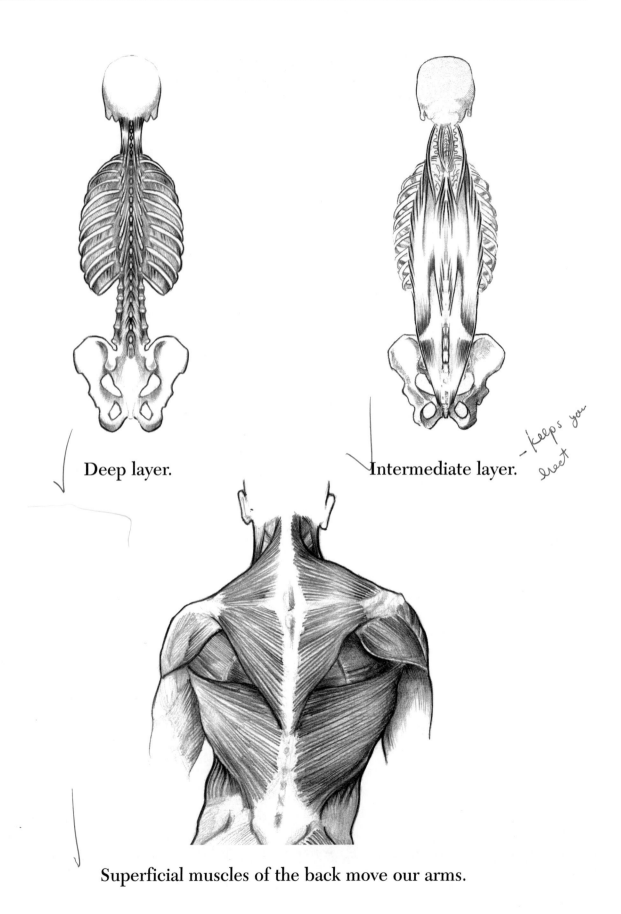

Deep layer.

Intermediate layer. — keeps you erect

Superficial muscles of the back move our arms.

But most people, when they think of "back muscles," do not think of the postural muscles I have just described. They think instead of the superficial muscles shown in the third picture. As the picture shows, the back presents a broad expanse of superficial muscles, including some quite large ones, and some with familiar names: trapezius, latissimus dorsi, deltoid. If a person undertakes a back workout at the gym, these are the muscles exercised. But consider what the exercises consist of. Lat pull-downs to exercise the latissumus dorsi, shrugging motions to exercise the trapezius, and so on. These may be back exercises, but all of them are performed with the *arms*. In other words, we exercise our backs by moving our arms. All the muscles shown in the third picture attach to the shoulder blade, collarbone, or humerus (some to more than one of those), which are parts of the arm. When we notice this we can understand that although the muscles usually thought of as "back muscles" are located on the back, with regard to function they are *arm* muscles.

Similar remarks apply to the chest muscles. These also are really arm muscles. That is, they move the arms even though they are situated on the chest. Once again, consider the exercises done by someone who wants to develop chest muscles: bench press, flies, and so on—all these are performed by moving the arms.

Having so many arm muscles on our backs and chests makes perfect sense when we bear two principles in mind. First, if the articulation of the bones at a joint permits many kinds of motion, many muscles will be needed to bring about the different motions. The shoulder joint is an exceptionally mobile joint, consequently many muscles are required to move the humerus in all its myriad ways. Second, in order to move a bone, a muscle must cross over a joint and attach to the bone it is moving. That means that the muscles that move the humerus must be situated on our backs and chests. They extend across the glenohumeral joint to attach to the humerus. In addition to the muscles that move the humerus, there are other muscles, also situated on the back and chest, that move the collarbone and shoulder blade. Those structures, like the humerus, can move in many ways, and their varied movements require many muscles.

A person who stands and sits in balance is supported in an upright position by the spine, which receives assistance in bending, in departing from and returning to balance, from the deep postural muscles of the back. That leaves the superficial muscles free to move the arms, which is their proper function. But this arrangement of different muscles doing their appropriate tasks can be compromised, particularly by downward pull or the misuse that is brought about and encouraged by the Posture Myths. Pushing "shoulders back," thrusting the "chest out" and doing the other things demanded by the Posture Myths—all these are accomplished with arm muscles that have been co-opted in the name of "posture." Back-oriented sitting, a common habit among pianists, involves constant tension of the arm muscles. Sometimes it leads to back, shoulder, and arm pain (also common among pianists). But whether there is pain or not, the arms obviously cannot move freely at the piano if there is underlying tension. If a person sits in a back-oriented way, free movement will be compromised and the playing will not be as good as it could be.

Innumerable movements used in piano playing are accomplished by muscles in the back and chest. For example, our elbows move constantly in playing, both toward and away from the keyboard and out to the sides and back. But every time the elbow moves, that motion occurs at the shoulder joint, perhaps the sterno-clavicular joint as well, and is caused by one or more of the "back" or "chest" muscles. If they are stiff or stretched or contracted, as they are for many pianists, motion will not be as free as it ought to be.

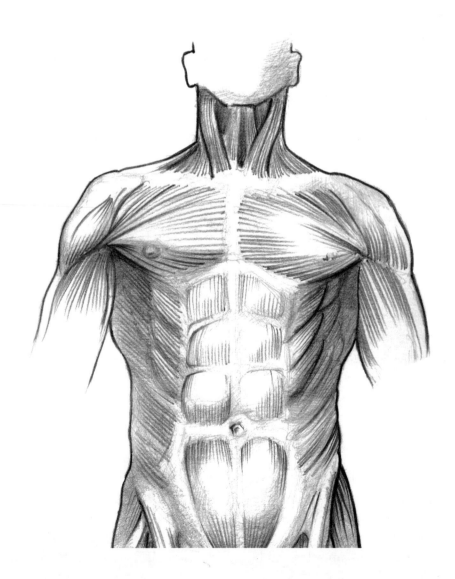

Like back muscles, the chest muscles move our arms.

[handwritten margin note top: But this can cause tension. Try to play in relaxed position, w/o constant stretching]

[handwritten margin note right: Bad =]

It is very easy for pianists to fall into habits of tension in muscles of the back, chest, and shoulder area. These are piano-playing muscles, since they move the arms, but it's easy not to be aware of them while we play the piano since, as pointed out earlier, we generally are aware of movement, not the muscles that cause the movement. Therefore, the muscles may be tense, but we don't notice because we're not aware of them in the first place. Any tendency to be unaware of tension will be reinforced if there is a habit of dis-embodiment. Furthermore, people who have absorbed the Posture Myths will have constant tension just from standing or sitting upright. They may be so accus-tomed to the tension that they do not notice it as such. They do not know they are tense because they do not know what it feels like not to be tense. Fortunately, all of these problems can be solved. When we learn to sit and stand in balance and include our entire arm structure in our body map we can develop new habits of free, painless movement at the piano.

༄

THE HAND

Most of the muscles that move the hand (the metacarpals) and fingers (the pha-langes) are in the forearm, not in the fin-gers.[1] There are no muscles in the fingers, although the small muscles in the hand do

---

[1] For convenience in this discussion I am using "fingers" in the ordinary way, according to which the fingers end at the main knuckle (MCP joint) and the "hand" is separate from the fingers. I am not speaking in the way I earlier advocat-ed, according to which the fingers extend all the way to the wrist bones, though that way of speaking is better from a movement point of view.

reach across the MCP joint to spread the fingers, bring them back together, and bend them at the MCP joint (these are the *interosseous* or "between the bones" mus-cles, which lie between the metacarpals). Hand muscles also contribute to move-ment of the thumb. But most movements of the hand and fingers are accomplished by muscles in the forearm.

That there are no muscles in the fingers comes as a surprise to most pianists. But it is not surprising that we should be more aware of our fingers than we are of the muscles that move them. Our kinesthetic sense receptors are designed to inform us of movement, not the causes of movement. Nevertheless, the fact that the muscles that move the fingers are distant from the fingers is very important.

The muscles of the forearm can be divided into two groups: the flexor muscles, which are on the palm (or ventral) side of the forearm, and the extensor muscles, which are on the other (dorsal) side. The flexors bend the fingers and hand downward (toward the palm); the extensors straight-en and lift the fingers and hand. Since the two sets of muscles bring about opposite movements, they are called opposing muscles. When the hand and fingers are moved in one direction by one set of muscles, the opposing muscles must release to permit easy motion. If the opposing muscles do not release, then the two muscle groups are working against each other. This is called *co-contraction*. Excessive co-contraction makes movement more difficult and can be a cause of injury.

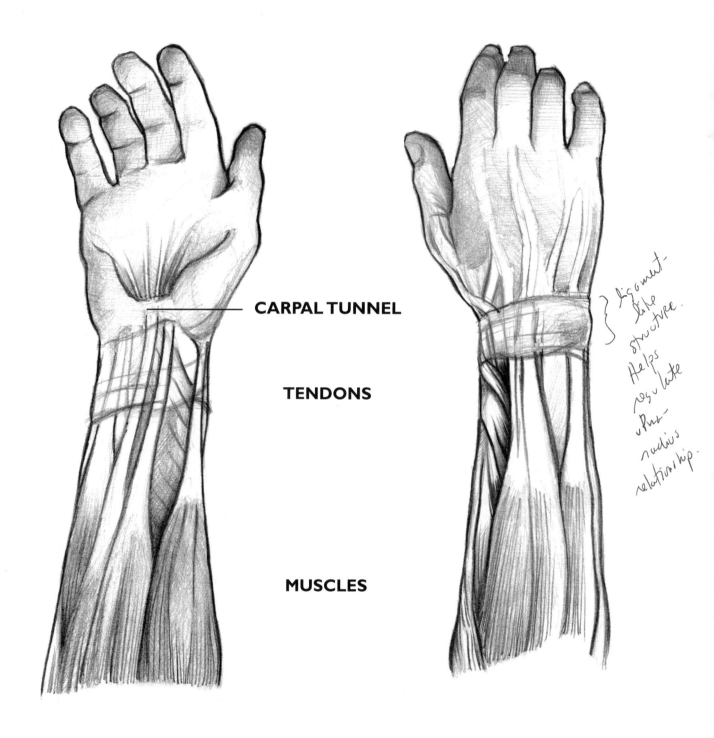

CARPAL TUNNEL

TENDONS

MUSCLES

} ligament-
like
structure.
Helps
regulate
ulnar-
radius
relationship.

Flexor muscles in the forearm
move the hand and fingers
toward the palm.

Extensor muscles in the forearm
straighten the fingers
and lift the hand.

The muscles that flex and extend the fingers are in the back of the forearm, far from the fingers they move. They connect to the fingers by long tendons that pass over the wrist and hand to the fingers. The tendons move back and forth as the muscles contract to move the fingers. Moving with the hand in extreme positions can put extra stress on the tendons, since the tendons must then follow a tortuous path to reach the part moved. This may result in less power delivered to the part, or in stress to the tendon as it rubs against neighboring structures.

Each joint of the fingers—each phalangeal joint—is bent by a different muscle. The first (MCP) joint, which joins the fingers to the hand, is moved by small muscles in the hand (interosseous muscles). The middle (PIP) joint is bent by muscles in the forearm (superficial flexor muscles). The end (DIP) joint of the fingers is also bent by muscles in the forearm (deep flexor muscles) which are closer to the forearm bones than the superficial flexor muscles.

☙

CURLED FINGERS

If we allow our hands to hang freely at our sides, the fingers assume a slightly curved position. I shall call this the "natural curve." This is the position in which muscles are not working either to straighten the fingers or to curl them. It is neutral for the fingers, the place from which motion is easiest. This is the appropriate base position for the fingers in piano playing. Sometimes pianists bend the two end joints of the fingers more acutely, producing a more pronounced curve than the natural one. I shall call this

"curled" fingers, and if it is chronic it is potentially injurious.

The reason chronically curled fingers can be dangerous is that curling the two end joints of the fingers is accomplished by contracting the flexor muscles on the lower side of the forearm. Lifting the fingers is accomplished by contracting the extensor muscles on the top of the forearm. Therefore, if I lift my fingers while maintaining the "curl" of the two end joints, I am using flexor muscles in active opposition to extensor muscles, a situation of co-contraction.

Co-contraction makes movement more difficult. Try moving your fingers up and down while keeping the two end joints curled. Then permit your fingers to release to the natural curve and move them up and down from the MCP joint. Moving them up and down in the natural curve is easier and faster than moving them up and down when holding them curled. Co-contraction is one of the causes of injury described in Chapter 9 of this book, and there are pianists who have suffered injury from playing with tightly curled fingers.

True.

Chronically curled fingers at the piano also encourage a shortening and tightening of the wrist. The wrist tends to assume the look of a hinge, instead of being the long, flexible structure described in the section on the wrist.

Nevertheless, playing with curled fingers is not only tolerated, it is advocated by some piano methods. There are even beginning methods that tell students to use a pencil to line up the tips of the fingers into a straight line—a recipe for co-contraction and shortening across the wrist. If a student practices diligently with the fingers held in that configuration, no one should be surprised if injury is the result. Some pianists keep their fingers curled in order to avoid having them extend over the black keys. Pianists and teachers should learn to resist any suggestion that the fingers be chronically held more tightly curled than the natural curve.

I am not saying that we can never curl our fingers safely at the piano. Some pianists do avoid curling, and use the natural curve almost exclusively. But we can move our fingers safely in many ways, including curling them if we wish, provided we release them again to the natural curve. The absence of release is what is dangerous. Some pianists court injury not because they curl their fingers at the moment of playing, which can be safe, but because they hold the non-playing fingers stiffly curled or stretched out to the side. Releasing the fingers is essential for injury-free playing.

THUMB ORIENTATION AND ULNAR DEVIATION

We saw earlier that thumb orientation, a mismapping of the rotation of the forearm, is one of the most common causes of pianists' injuries. Understanding the location and relationship of the muscles that move the hand makes clear why thumb orientation is so harmful in all activities, not just piano playing.

Very often, thumb-oriented movement gives a characteristic appearance to the hand. The hand is persistently turned sideways, to a position of ulnar deviation. Because of this, chronic ulnar deviation is usually a reliable indication of thumb orientation. However, we must bear in mind that ulnar deviation refers to a position of the hand whereas thumb orientation refers to a way of organizing movement, not to a position. Very often, when the hand assumes an ulnar-deviated position, the movement used to assume the position is a thumb-oriented movement. However, it is also possible for the hand to move into an ulnar-deviated position but to do so freely, without thumb orientation. If that happens, the position is benign since there is no tension. There are some electric bass players whose technique obliges them to play in a position of ulnar deviation. Those who adopt the position in a thumb-oriented manner become injured; those who adopt the same position without thumb orientation do not.

We know that anatomically the ulna is stable in forearm rotation and the radius moves across it. But in thumb orientation, movement is organized around the radius instead. That is, the person's body map represents movement organized around the radius and so the person attempts to stabilize the radius to make *it* the axis. Now, the muscles that rotate the forearm are the deepest muscles in the forearm— right next to the bones. When the forearm rotates freely, those deep muscles are activated; the superficial muscles of the forearm are not involved, so they can be loose. In thumb orientation, however, the attempt to stabilize the radius is accomplished by tensing those superficial muscles. Chronically thumb-oriented people have tension in the superficial muscles of the forearm.

But the superficial muscles of the forearm are the muscles that move the fingers. If a pianist is thumb oriented, those muscles and their tendons are continually tense just from the action of stabilizing the radius, instead of being available for easy movement of the fingers. As a result, finger movements become more difficult—that is, the muscles have to work harder to produce a given movement, which puts additional stress on the tendons. We have a situation of potential injury. When the person corrects the body map to make it fit the anatomical facts, movement can become little finger and ulna oriented.

You can experience the difference this makes. With your little finger roughly in line with your ulna, move your fingers rapidly up and down from the MCP joints. They move easily. Now adopt a thumb-oriented movement: deviate your hand toward the little finger (ulnar deviation), and as you do so, feel that you are simultaneously thrusting your thumb strongly forward. In that position, try moving your fingers. Most likely, you will find that they do not move as easily as before.

Also characteristic of thumb orientation is a sense that the little finger is weak. In fact, the fourth and fifth fingers are not weak, but they feel weak if they are used without proper support from the arm. When a pianist develops a habit of little finger orientation and uses appropriate arm movements toward and away from the fallboard to adjust for the different lengths of the fingers, the fourth and fifth fingers feel as strong as the other fingers.

(These movements require freedom of the shoulder joint.)

Some pianistic tasks that many pianists accomplish by using ulnar deviation are: bringing the thumb to a black key, bringing the thumb to a white key in white-key passages, and playing octaves with 1 and 4 or 1 and 3. Playing white keys while preventing the long fingers from extending over the black keys may also encourage ulnar deviation. The mere position of ulnar deviation is not harmful in itself, but if deviation from neutral is sustained or frequent, the pianist may easily develop a chronic habit of thumb orientation. Some pianists chronically hold the upper arm far out from the body, which encourages ulnar deviation. Most pianists who use a lot of ulnar deviation do so in a thumb-oriented way. Since the situations mentioned above arise frequently in piano playing, you should attend meticulously to the way you accomplish them and make certain that you establish a secure habit of little finger orientation. Ulnar deviation is not necessary for the tasks mentioned; some pianists develop a technique that uses almost no ulnar deviation.

Many people are thumb oriented in daily life as well as at the piano. A person whose habits involve tension at the piano cannot change those habits at the piano only. Watch for thumb orientation as you reach for doorknobs or faucets, as you open your car door, as you reach to pick up a plate. You can use those other activities as opportunities to observe and correct your body map. When the body map is accurate and adequate, new habits of movement will inform all life activities.

THE FOREARM ARCH

When we stand in balance with awareness of the support of our bony structure, we can discover a sense of "connectedness" from our feet up through the entire core of the body. Some people describe this as being "grounded" or "centered" and attribute it to a balanced organization that supports us through optimal alignment aided by postural reflexes.

A similar thing can happen in relation to our arms. Obviously, we do not stand on our hands at the piano, nor do our hands support our weight. Nevertheless, we can develop an awareness of an organization in our arms and hands that is analogous to the sense of being organized around our core when we stand in balance. A good place to start to cultivate this awareness is the arch of the hand and forearm.

Geometrically, an arch is a remarkably stable, efficient structure for support and weight delivery. When its keystone is in place, the arch is self-supporting. Some stone arches constructed in ancient times without use of mortar are still standing and bearing weight after thousands of years. We have seen that our bodies exploit the geometry of the arch in several places, notably the arches of the pelvis and the foot. The forearm does not present a rigid arch like the arch of the pelvis. But when the bones of the fingers, wrist, and forearm are aligned as in the illustration on p. 111, their geometry is analogous to an arch and confers some of the same mechanical advantage.

KEYSTONE

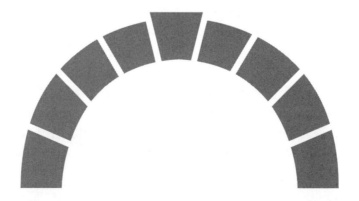

The geometry of the arch makes it an exceptionally efficient, strong, and stable structure.

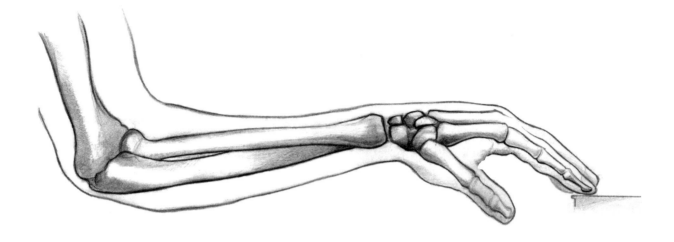

The arch of the hand and forearm can be the basis of playing without tension, yet with ease, control, and power.

You can learn to experience the arch this way: first, stand in balance with your arms hanging freely at your sides. Your fingers, hand, and forearm naturally tend to assume the arch shape: fingers are bent in the natural curve, the wrist is approximately straight, and the hand is not thumb oriented. Without changing any of that alignment, think of it as an arch. The fingertips and the elbow represent opposite ends of the arch and the metacarpal bone is the keystone. Now, still keeping the arch exactly intact, you can bend at the elbow and move the arch up and down. Fingers, wrist, and forearm all move together.

Now take that to the piano. Sit at the piano with the bench adjusted so that the tip of the elbow is even with the top of the white keys. Moving principally at the elbow joint

and still keeping the arch in mind, let the arch descend so that one finger lands on a piano key. Notice how that feels. There should not be even the slightest "collapse" in the wrist or any other joint as you depress the key, nor should the fingers or hand anticipate the movement of the arm. It helps to think of the metacarpal bone as the keystone of the arch. When the arch comes down, bringing the finger with it to depress the key, the sensation is that the "keystone" holds the whole structure in place with no muscular effort.

The sensation of depressing a key this way comes as a revelation to pianists who experience it for the first time. There is a sense of effortlessness combined with perfect security and great control; the forearm arch feels self-supporting yet it stands securely on the key. When you

111

move the fingers, hand, and forearm with a sense of the arch organization, you will discover an immediate improvement in tone and better control of volume as compared to other ways of playing. The arch structure represents a position of mechanical advantage in relation to the piano and it can become the basis of a non-injurious technique.

One reason the arch works so well is that it discourages thumb orientation. With the arch organization, the power needed to depress the keys is delivered to the piano through the bony structure, much the way weight is supported and delivered through the bony structure when we stand or sit. Movement is organized around the structure, not based on tensing muscles. Muscles do not have to work as hard. We saw earlier that thumb orientation involves tensing muscles to stabilize the radius. With movement organized around the bony structure, stability is achieved without tension. The muscles can release. It is similar to the way support through the core of the torso permits the release of back and chest muscles.

The forearm arch goes from the elbow to the fingertip, but it is part of a whole arm that includes the humerus, collarbone, and shoulder blade in addition to the arch. When all these parts of the arm are integrated in awareness, the arms can feel unified, powerful, free to move, and yet not heavy. There can be a feeling of connectedness that extends from the fingertip all the way to the core support of the body. This is sometimes described as "support from the core" for the arms. Cultivating this sense of connectedness

improves the quality of movement and the playing.

In using the image of an arch I am not advocating that the forearm *appear* highly arched; I am not endorsing over-arching. The forearm appears to be approximately level. (That is partly because the descent of the arch in back, from the apex at the metacarpal bone to the lowest point of the tip of the ulna, is masked by forearm muscles.) Once you have grasped the concept of alignment through the bony structure and experienced the stability it confers, you should think of the arch not as a visual image but rather a structural, kinesthetic sensation. Notice also that the shape of the arch is not fixed or rigid; it adjusts for different pianistic situations. In playing chords and octaves, for example, the wrist is higher than it is in single-note playing, but there can still be a sense of support through the bony structure.

SUSPENSION OF THE ARMS

The arms are not supported by our core in the same way the head is. The head sits on top of the spine like a gazing ball on a pedestal, delivering its weight directly to a structure designed to receive the weight. Our arms are not like that. They do not rest on anything. The shoulder blades do not attach to the ribs nor do they rest on them (which is just as well since the ribs must move and are not designed to receive weight). The collarbone likewise does not attach to the ribs or rest on them. It attaches to the breastbone, but it merely anchors there—it does not deliver weight to the breastbone (which is no more designed to receive weight than the ribs are). Rather than *resting* on a support, the arms are *suspended* out to the sides, over the core of the body. The analogy of a suspension bridge can be illuminating. Consider the central part (the part in black) of the bridge shown below:

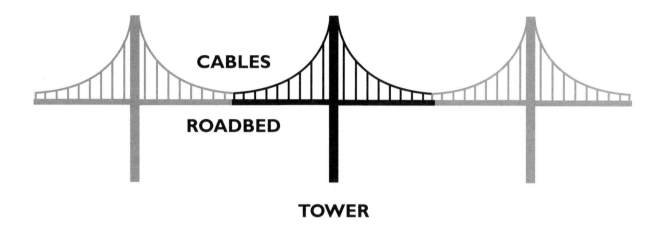

The vertical tower supports the whole structure. It bears the weight of the structure and delivers it to the ground. But although the tower supports the roadbed, the roadbed does not *rest* on the tower or on anything else. The roadbed is supported by the cables—that is, it is *suspended* from the tower by means of the cables.

Our arms are analogously suspended from our core support, but they differ from the roadbed in being mobile in various ways. So imagine a more complex suspension bridge with cables below the roadbed as well as above.

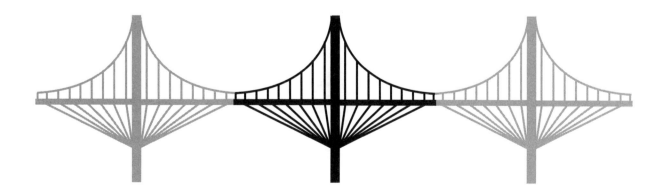

Tension on the cables below would move the roadbed lower, provided the upper cables could stretch by the proper amount. Similarly, tension on the upper cables would lift the roadbed, provided the lower cables could stretch. In this way, the roadbed can move up and down. Nevertheless, we can imagine that there is a position of approximate equilibrium where all the cables support the roadbed in such a way that tension on any one cable is minimal. Our arms are similar in principle (but more complex because they can move forward and back as well as up and down, and they can rotate).

Look now at the superficial muscles of the back and chest with this image in mind.

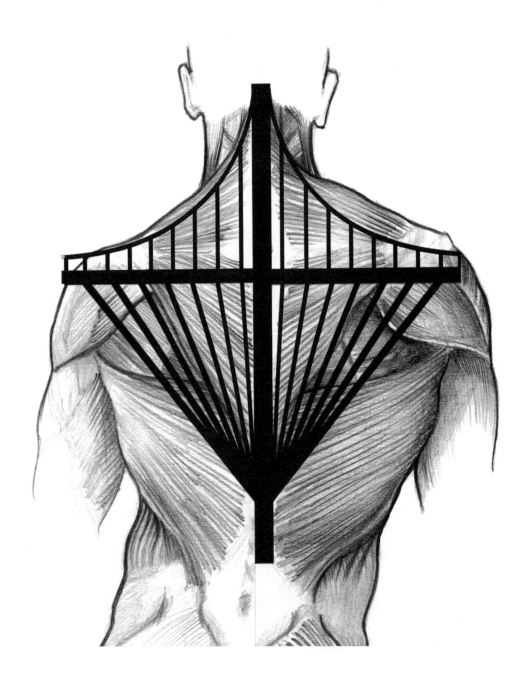

When the arms are properly balanced and suspended out to the sides, tension on muscles is minimal and the arm structure is free to move. On the other hand, if a person has a habit such that the resting position of the arms is lower or higher than or forward or back of the balanced position, then some muscle or muscle group is *pulling* the arm out of equilibrium. At the same time, some other muscle or muscle group must stretch in order to accommodate the arm's being out of equilibrium. In other words, chronic departure from the position of equilibrium represents chronic tension of some arm muscles, chronic stretching of others. The person's piano playing will be less free (and consequently worse) than it could be. This is not something to be taken lightly or dismissed. Remember that if imbalance of the arm structure is chronic (as it is for many pianists) then tension will be present *before the first key is depressed* and the playing of *every single note* will require some compensation for the underlying tension.

If the tower of our suspension bridge could feel things, we can suppose that it would be aware of weight delivered through the core to the ground, but not aware of one cable more than another since the cables (by hypothesis) are in equilibrium with minimal tension on each. If any one cable became tense we can imagine that the tension would distract or dilute the tower's awareness of the central core support.

If the bridge were to use the lower cables to pull the roadbed down, the way humans use muscles to pull their arms down, there would be a moving *down* of the roadbed accompanied by a pull *upward* on the tower where the cables that pull the roadbed down attach to the base of the tower. This upward tension, I am supposing, would detract from the tower's awareness of a unified delivery of weight downward to the ground.

Now imagine that the cables pulling down on the roadbed are suddenly released. The roadbed will *rise*. What the tower will experience is a sense of lightness and release in the roadbed. It will simultaneously feel a more direct and unified *downward* vertical delivery of weight, since the cables tugging upward on the base of the tower have been released. Thus, the roadbed feels *lighter* and at the same time the sense of support through the core of the tower is more vivid and unified.

That is exactly how it feels in our body as we learn to release our arms (which depends on learning to release the head on the spine). The arms are not supported in the sense of resting *on* anything. Instead they "float" or "are suspended," but their liberation heightens our sense of a unified support through our core. In this way it makes sense to speak of "support through the core" for the arms. Conversely, awareness of a tightening in the core—or a restriction in the awareness of weight freely delivered through the core—may indicate tension in the arms, that is, in the muscles that are usually called "back muscles" but which are really arm muscles. Release that tension by renewing the sense of support through the core and the arms will move more easily. Piano playing improves.

With this image of the suspension of the arm structure in mind, pianists should review the procedure described earlier, in the section on balance of the arm structure, whose purpose was to help the arms learn to find the place of optimal balance (p. 75). We can now think of that place of balance as the place where the arm structure is suspended in equilibrium and the arms are free to move.

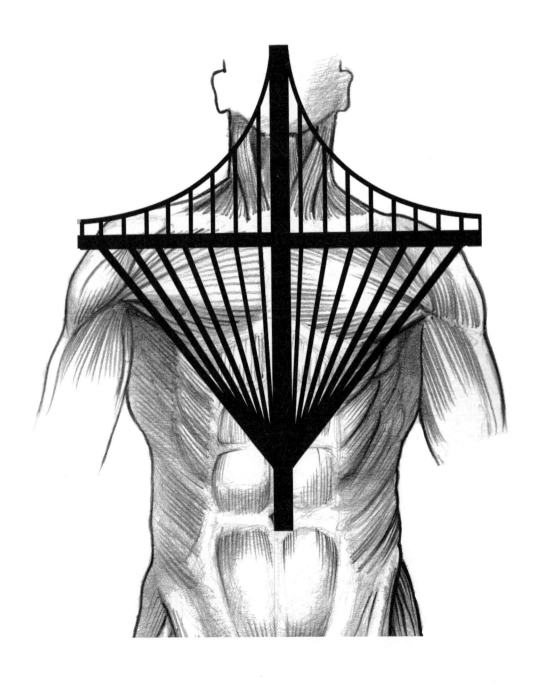

Comparing the support for the arms to a suspension bridge is a simplification, but it is accurate enough to be useful in helping us to move better. The actual structure and organization of the arm structure is far more complex. As currently understood, the suspension of the collarbone and shoulder blade (and thereby the whole arm) over the ribs appears to come from several interrelated factors: the bones' shape, the interplay of connective tissue, and involuntary postural patterns that support or buoy up voluntary movement.

These involuntary postural patterns, like the one that gives a sense of a spring in our step, are currently being studied and described by scientists. Perhaps in time they will be as well understood as circulation of the blood now is. In the meantime, we who cannot study them experimentally can study them experientially as we find the balance and use of the collarbones and shoulder blades that allows us to feel continually buoyed up and fluid in our upper torsos, enhancing the quality of our playing.

CHAPTER 6: MAPPING BREATHING

If we are alive, we are breathing. We breathe all the time, awake and asleep, at the piano and away from it. Since breathing is automatic and occurs whether we are aware of it or not, pianists may think they can leave breathing to take care of itself. Why pay attention to something that will happen anyway, when we have so many other things to think about?

In fact, many pianists have problems related to breathing. Some hold their breath while they play. Others are afraid to take a deep breath out of fear that the act of breathing will disturb what they are doing at the piano. Sometimes they are right. Taking a deep breath, the way they do it, *does* disturb their playing. Some of the most common breathing problems for pianists are caused by:

1. Trying to get air into the belly.
2. Tightening the abdominal wall.
3. Trying to expand the chest forwards.
4. Trying to use chest muscles for breathing.
5. Tightening the muscles in the throat.
6. Creating tension in the name of "diaphragmatic breathing."
7. Breathing as if the windpipe were behind the esophagus instead of in front of it.
8. Trying to breathe from bottom to top (imagining that the lungs fill from the bottom like a pitcher).

All these problems can be regarded as mapping errors. They affect piano playing because trying to breathe in accordance with the faulty map creates tension that inhibits the free use of the arms. The problems are solved by correctly mapping the structure and movement of breathing. Let us summarize the facts.[1]

&

LOCATION OF THE LUNGS

The lungs are in the upper third of the torso and occupy the upper half of the thorax or rib area. The top of each lung is higher than most people think—just above the collarbone. The bottom of the lung in front is approximately even with the bottom of the breastbone. The lungs do not only occupy the front part of the chest, they also extend out to the sides and back. If you stand or sit with awareness of your core support, you should think of your lungs *alongside* and *behind* your core support (not just filling the space in front of your core support). Because the lungs are high up in the body, air travels only a short distance to reach them. And because the lungs occupy the sides and back as well as the front of the thoracic cavity, their capacity is quite large.

---

[1] Although the information about breathing presented here is sufficient for pianists, it is not sufficient for wind players or singers or pianists who accompany their own singing. Those musicians need a more detailed map.

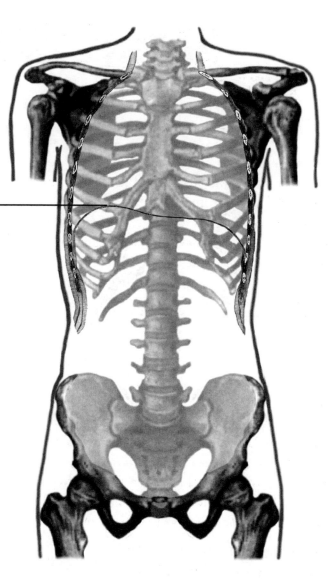

THE LUNGS

Occupy the upper part of the rib area, above the diaphragm.

DIAPHRAGM

The abdominal cavity contains organs of digestion and other structures. Air does not go here.

Muscles of the pelvic cavity support breathing.

BACK

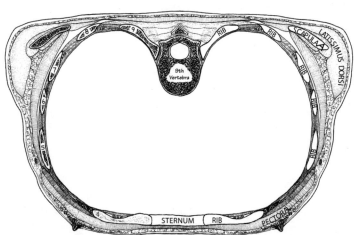

The weight-bearing spine is inside the ribs. The lungs occupy space on both sides of the weight-bearing spine, as well as in front of it and behind it.

FRONT

❧
MOVEMENT OF BREATHING

In principle, breathing is simple: movement of the ribs and diaphragm causes the space in the thoracic cavity to become alternately larger and smaller. As the space gets larger or smaller, air goes in or out.

The ribs attach to the spine at joints that allow movement up and down. From the spine, the ribs circle around to the front where they attach to flexible cartilage which connects to the breastbone. With joints in back and flexible cartilage in front, the ribs are capable of movement at both ends. Movement of the ribs is accomplished by the *intercostal* ("between the ribs") muscles. These muscles cause the arc of each rib to swing upwards and downwards, like a bucket handle. As each rib swings upward, its center moves further out to the side, enlarging the space in the thoracic cavity. Air flows into the larger space. When the ribs descend, the space becomes smaller and air flows out again.

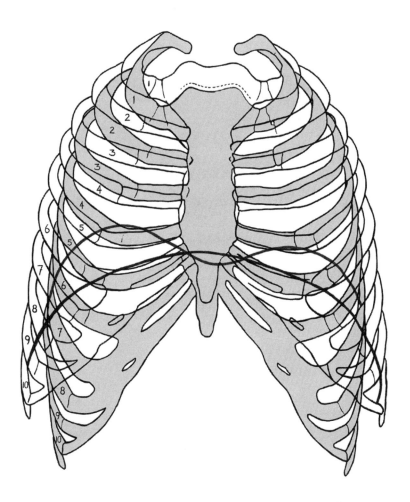

On inhalation, all the ribs move up and out.
On exhalation, they move down and in.

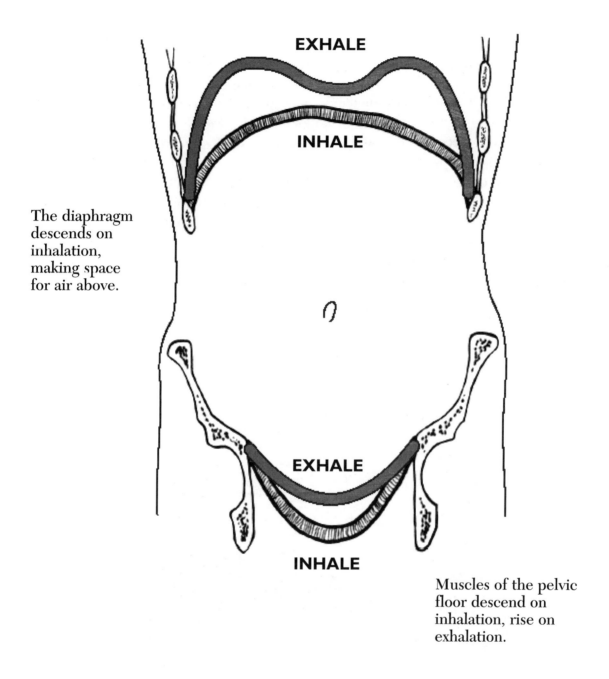

EXHALE

INHALE

The diaphragm descends on inhalation, making space for air above.

EXHALE

INHALE

Muscles of the pelvic floor descend on inhalation, rise on exhalation.

The diaphragm is a large dome-shaped muscle under the lungs that separates the upper rib area, which contains the heart and lungs, from the lower rib area, which contains the stomach, spleen, and liver (further down, in the lower torso, are the intestines and other organs). When the diaphragm contracts, it moves from being highly dome-shaped to being less dome-shaped and its diameter increases. This movement enlarges the space above the diaphragm, and air flows into the space. When the diaphragm rises again to its highly domed shape, air flows out.

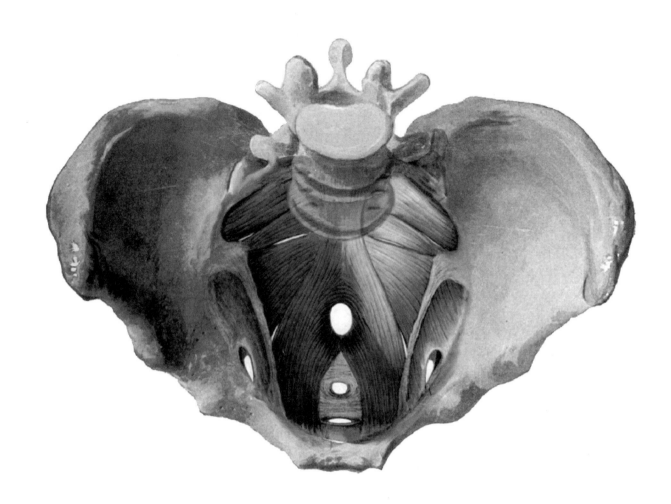

Muscles of the pelvic floor support breathing.
Freedom of these muscles is also vital for
proper balance on the bench.

The descent of the diaphragm, which creates more space for air above the diaphragm, simultaneously reduces the space below the diaphragm where the stomach, liver, and other organs are. Those structures are moved out of the way by the descending diaphragm. Therefore, the descent of the diaphragm is accompanied by a proportional widening of the torso below the diaphragm and a descent of the pelvic floor.

Unfortunately, many people develop habits that inhibit breathing. They may also have wrong ideas about how breathing is accomplished. Some of the wrong ideas are created or encouraged by the Posture Myths.

The same people who tell you to "stand up straight, shoulders back, chest out, stomach in," etc. are likely to tell you that in taking a deep breath the chest expands forwards. It is quite true that there is a natural deepening of the chest that comes from the combination of rib movement and movement of the breastbone. In that sense, the chest does expand forward, and the movement is appropriate. But people who talk of expanding their chests usually have in mind something more active, and they actively thrust their chests forward. What they are really doing is hoisting up the entire thorax and thrusting it forward. That is a *spinal* movement. It is pointless as far as breathing is concerned since it does not increase the space for air, and it is damaging to piano playing since it is accomplished by tensing the muscles of our backs, inhibiting free movement of the arms. A pianist whose body map makes breathing a matter of thrusting the chest outward will indeed find that breathing interferes with piano playing and may be afraid to take a deep breath, or may try to hold the breath or breathe shallowly.

Trying to use chest muscles for breathing likewise inhibits free movement of the arms. Many of the muscles located on our backs and chest actually serve to move our arms (see the chapter on muscles), which is why enlisting them to serve a misguided conception of breathing inhibits movement of the arms and detracts from piano playing.

Another harmful habit is to tense the stomach muscles while inhaling. Some people believe you should "suck in your gut" as you inhale. But flattening your stomach by tensing the abdominal muscles prevents the natural widening of the lower torso caused by the diaphragm contracting in normal breathing. With abdominal muscles tense, there is no space below for the diaphragm to descend and therefore less space above the diaphragm for air.

If a person maps the arms as resting on the ribs, breathing will be inhibited, as will free movement of the arms in piano playing (see the section on support for the arms). Imbalance in the torso, caused by slumping or trying to maintain "good posture," constricts movement of the ribs in breathing and also reduces mobility of the arms.

In describing the movement of breathing I have not mentioned activity in the neck and throat. Many people think that when they breathe they are sucking air in with their throats. This is a fantasy. We can't suck air in with our throats because there are no muscles there that can do it. People with this mapping error tense their throats, which causes breathing to be noisy. Noisy breathing may be a reason why some pianists try to hold their breath. Holding the breath is a bad solution. The proper solution is to correct the body map so that breathing is silent, effortless, and automatic, and then experiment with different ways of relating breathing to piano playing.

Pay attention to your ribs and notice them moving up and out to the sides. Let them move up and out with no involvement whatsoever of your neck and throat. Air is going in and out of the lungs, and if the neck and throat are free there is no noise. Do not tighten your abdominal muscles or resist the natural widening of the lower torso as the diaphragm descends. Some people are so accustomed to tension in their necks when they breathe that when they first free their necks and feel their ribs moving they cannot believe that air is going in and out. But it is, and they can learn to sense the quiet movement of the air.

ॐ

BREATHING WITH THE PHRASE

Singers and wind players have no choice: they must coordinate their breathing with the phrasing of the music. Pianists, however, are free to choose. Pianists can coordinate breathing with phrasing if they find it convenient or effective, but they are not obliged to do that. They may choose to breathe as they would in any other activity, allowing the body automatically to meet its need for air. Or they can switch back and forth. Some pianists breathe independent of musical phrasing when playing solo literature, but when accompanying singers and wind players they coordinate their breathing with the musical phrase, as the singer or wind player does. They say this helps the ensemble.

Pianists can choose to breathe with the phrase or not, or to switch back and forth. Which choice they make does not matter, but they must make a choice. Otherwise, breathing feels at odds with the music, which can lead to a lot of tension. Once breathing is properly mapped and the choice is made, breathing and piano playing are coordinated.

CHAPTER 7: MAPPING THE PIANO

❧
THE PIANO MAP

The body map is the representation in the brain that governs movement. But this book is not about mere bodily movement, it is about movement directed to an end—the creation of music at the piano. As we know, how I move my arm depends on how I think of the structure of my arm. How I move my arm *at the piano* depends on that, but also on how I think my arm and hand interact with the piano to produce music. How we think of the piano affects the way we move at the piano.

The representation of how our body interacts with the piano is what I shall call our "piano map." Like our body map, our piano map can be accurate or inaccurate, adequate or inadequate, conscious or unconscious. Since we move our bodies to play the piano, our piano map has to include our body map; all the information about the body offered in this book is—or should be— part of our piano map. However, a good piano map also requires information about the piano.[1]

The modern piano is a complex, ingenious, remarkably responsive mechanical device that converts kinetic energy— motion—into sound. Piano sound comes from the vibration of metal wires, called strings. The strings are caused to vibrate by being hit by felt-covered hammers; there is one hammer for each key of the piano. Depressing a key moves a series of levers, which activate the hammer and *throw* it toward the strings. The hammer hits the string, causing it to vibrate, and instantly rebounds. All the energy that produces the sound is transferred at the instant the hammer hits the string (unlike a voice or a cello, where energy can be continuously supplied to sustain the tone).

Each string is tuned to a definite pitch, the fundamental tone for that string, but in addition to vibrating along its entire length to produce the fundamental tone, the string also vibrates in segments, producing a mix of overtones. Therefore, the sound from a piano string is not a simple tone of one frequency, but a complex sound.

The facts just summarized relate to the inner workings of the piano. Of course, when we play the piano we touch the keys, not the hammers, strings, and action. We need to know about them, however, because of their bearing on the way our fingers interact with the keys.

---

[1] In what follows I discuss the piano, not the harpsichord, clavichord, or other keyboard instruments. Players of other instruments need to determine what facts about their instrument need to be in their harpsichord map, clavichord map, etc. Although our piano map includes our body map along with facts about the piano, that does not mean that we "become one" with the piano. We interact with the piano, we do not unite with it.

✣
MAPPING THE POINT OF SOUND

If you slowly depress a key, you will feel a point of slight resistance, a "bump," shortly before the key reaches the keybed. That bump corresponds to the activation of the escapement mechanism in the action. It is the point at which the hammer is thrown toward the string, momentarily losing contact with the rest of the action. Using the terminology of Dorothy Taubman, I shall call it the "point of sound." Pianists need to map several things about the point of sound.

Sound is caused by the hammer being thrown against the string as the key passes the point of sound. Now, the key reaches the point of sound *before* it reaches the keybed. That is obvious, but it has important consequences. The first consequence is: nothing that happens *after* the key passes the point of sound can change or affect the sound, in particular, nothing that happens at the keybed. No amount of pressing, sliding, or wobbling on the keybed can alter a sound that has already been produced. What we do at the keybed does matter, because it may facilitate or impede motion to the *next* key, but it cannot affect a sound that is already in the air (though, of course, the finger can control the *length* of the sound by holding the key down to keep the damper off the string). Pressing down on the keybed, for example, perhaps in the name of improving the tone, is pointless. The sound can no longer be changed, so pressing down just represents unnecessary tension.

That the point of sound comes before the key reaches the keybed has another important consequence, namely that the volume and quality of the sound depend on the *velocity* of the key descent, *not on the amount of weight or force delivered to the keybed.* After all, at the instant the key reaches the point of sound there is no way for the piano to register the amount of force that is depressing the key. All the piano can respond to is how fast the key is descending; *the speed and only the speed* of the descent determines the speed of the hammer hitting the string, which in turn determines the volume and quality of the sound.

This point contradicts a lot of conventional pedagogical opinion and may seem surprising to some pianists. Many people talk, teach, and play as if the force or weight used to depress the key could affect the sound. To help counteract that view, and reinforce the conclusion of the last paragraph, I shall offer an analogy. Imagine yourself on the second story of a five-story building. You are seated, looking out the window. You can see outside but you cannot see the ground below your window. People on the different floors above are dropping various weights, which you can see falling past your window, although you cannot see them at the beginning of their fall, nor can you see them hit the ground. Since they are dropped from different heights, the weights pass your window with different velocities, and if you have an excellent eye you might learn to distinguish their velocities. But there is no way you could ascertain the force with which they are about to hit the ground. You don't know how much they weigh, only how fast they are going. One object might weigh five times as much as another object yet if they travel at the same speed they will seem alike to you at your window, even though, on impact, one of them makes a hole in the sidewalk and the other doesn't.[2] To you they are indistinguishable. The analogy I have offered is intended to give readers an image of a situation in which the velocity of a moving object, not its weight or momentum, triggers a response. In that particular way, the piano is like you at your window. Just as you respond to the velocities of the objects passing your window, not to the force with which they will hit the ground, so the piano activates the hammer in relation to the velocity of the key at the point of sound, not the amount of force that will, an instant later, arrive at the keybed.

As I pointed out above, changing the volume or quality of the sound must be accomplished by changing the speed of key descent, not by changing the amount of force on the keybed. It is possible to present the same point in another way, by considering how sound is produced on the piano. Sound is produced by the kinetic energy of the hammer being transferred to the string. Changing the sound requires changing the kinetic energy of the hammer. Now, the kinetic energy of the hammer is a function of its mass and velocity. But the mass of the hammer is constant. The only thing that can *change* from one occasion to the next is its velocity. Consequently, any changes in the volume and quality of the sound must come from changes in the velocity of the hammer, which is determined by the velocity of the key at the point of sound. There are no other possibilities.

Although this conclusion is inescapable, it may seem implausible at first. How can mere changes in the speed of the hammer

hitting the string give the immense variety of sounds that we hear from a well-played piano? Recall that the piano is remarkably responsive and that piano sound is complex, not simple. As the hammer goes faster, it imparts more energy to the string; as it goes slower, it imparts less energy. That alters the volume, as everyone knows. But volume of sound is not the only thing that changes: as the hammer goes faster or slower the mix of overtones shifts also, so the *quality* of the sound changes as well as the volume. As the hammer goes faster and faster, changes in volume become less striking than changes in quality; eventually the sound becomes, to most ears, harsher and uglier.

There is another vital point. As mentioned earlier, the kinetic energy delivered to the string is a function of the mass and the velocity of the hammer. But kinetic energy fluctuates not with the velocity but with the *square* of the velocity. Consequently, a change in velocity by a certain percent, say ten percent, will result in a *larger* change in the kinetic energy delivered to the string—twenty percent, perhaps. This means that *seemingly slight changes in the speed of key descent produce large differences in volume and tone quality.*[3]

---

[2] The point can also be put this way: you know the velocities of the objects but you do not know, nor can you determine, their momentum.

[3] This discussion has focused on changes in volume and quality of a single note. In real music, contrasts of tone quality and dynamics are not mainly based on comparing separate soundings of a single note, but on contrasts between different notes, played simultaneously or in succession. The pedals, both the damper pedal and the una corda pedal, also affect tone quality and dynamics. These things vastly expand the range of expressive possibilities in music, but do not alter the conclusions reached in the text.

The facts just presented need to be part of every pianist's piano map, since they affect the way we move at the piano and, consequently, the quality of our playing. To place them securely in your piano map, you need to cultivate an active awareness of your fingers interacting with the piano. Develop a vivid, tactile awareness of the finger in contact with the key. Note that the optimum point of contact is not the finger*tip* but slightly further back, more on the pad. One reason for this—there are several—is that the pad is a richer source of tactile information. Become aware of the distance the key descends. Feel your fingers in contact with the surface of the keys. Become aware of the point of sound. Let the ends of your fingers feel alive. With regard to *motion* the fingers are no more important than any other part of the body in playing the piano, but with regard to *perception* they are vital. They are the focus of our tactile awareness of the piano. Moreover, they not only touch the piano, they also receive *feedback* from the keys. You should regard them not just as carrying out the commands of the brain but as gathering information and sending it back to the brain and the rest of your body.

If you combine an acute tactile awareness of the fingers on the keys with a vivid kinesthetic awareness of your movement, you can learn to recognize and deliver the precise amount of work needed to obtain the sound you want. I have pointed out that pressure applied to the keybed does not alter a sound that has already been produced. But pressure on the keybed does influence movement to the next note. We do need to arrive at the keybed with a secure sense of contact and no "holding up" anywhere. This grounds us and enables movement to the next note, just as support from the floor enables our next step when we are walking. However, any additional force applied to the keybed merely inhibits movement.

Many pianists use excessive force, which is a serious cause of injury (see Chapter 9). It can also contribute to a harsh, inexpressive tone. The harsh tone does not come from the amount of force on the keybed but from the fact that a pianist who uses excessive force is likely to depress the key very fast, altering the mix of overtones and, consequently, the tone. That is: although force applied to the keybed does not affect the sound, the *intent* to arrive at the keybed a certain way or to apply force to the keybed may alter the way we approach the key—that is, the speed of key descent—thereby altering the tone and volume. A pianist who understands this, and understands that excessive force is a serious cause of injury, can learn to get a desired tone by controlling the key descent, with very little force directed into the keybed. Fantasies of "dropping weight" can be dangerous; the suggestion to "play as if the keybed were six inches lower" is especially harmful. Offered, I presume, in hope of obtaining a "big" sound, it is more likely to lead to a harsh sound and, in time, to injury. If you have a sense of your fingers being "stopped" by the keybed, chances are you are using excessive force. Someone who habitually uses excessive force will need to learn just how much force is really needed. At first it will seem like nothing.

❧
MAPPING LISTENING AND SPACE

Although the *moment* of sound production is when the key reaches the point of sound, the *location* of sound production is elsewhere: the place where sound is produced is the place where the hammer hits the string. That is where we should focus our listening. Direct your listening to the strings which make the sound, and to the place on the strings where the hammer hits. Your *tactile* focus is your fingers, but the focus of your *listening* is the actual sound, which comes from deep in the piano. Notice that tension in your face and neck interferes with listening.

Having mapped your body and your piano, you also need to map the space in which you play. By this I do not mean the physical room in which you sit, but the space you *play to,* the space you claim *in your music.* If the space you command in your playing is confined to your arms and hands and the piano keyboard, you will move differently from the way you move if you command a bigger space. Commanding a bigger space, your sound will be different, and more expressive. One helpful reminder is "Never practice in a space smaller than the smallest space in which you will ever perform." Another is to think "Whole body, whole piano, whole world." You may be sitting in a small practice room, but your music can include the earth and stars.

Mapping your listening and the space in which you play is much more important than the few sentences devoted to it in this book would suggest. However, its importance is not a matter of injury prevention. You will not develop pain in your arms from playing to a small space. What will happen, though, is artistically just as bad. You will risk joining the ranks of pianists who are not injured, who play all the notes but communicate none of the music, and leave their audience cold. Mapping the space in which we play is one of the things that makes our playing significant and communicative, transforming it from mere playing into an artistic activity.

CHAPTER 8: ADDITIONAL CONCERNS OF ORGANISTS

With very few exceptions, the material contained in this book is applicable to organists as well as pianists. Organists should read the book as though it were written for them, taking note of those inserts and comments directed to the specific needs and concerns organists have. In this chapter we will review and elaborate on the material organists need to know for free and easy playing. Reading this chapter is not a substitute for reading the entire book. It is simply intended as a quick review and as a practical aid in your journey toward properly mapping your body at the organ console.

MAPPING MOVEMENTS FOR ORGANISTS

It is assumed at this point that organists (and pianists) have read and understood enough to begin the process of properly mapping the body. Any improvements or corrections to the body map will lead to improvements in movement at the keyboard. But, organists, let us take a look at some critical and often problematic areas.

Movement of the Arm Structure

Organists must have the freedom to move their arms. That seems to be an obvious statement, but many organists suffer from a debilitating lack of mobility in the arm structure. Organists should read again that portion of this book devoted to mapping the joints of the arm structure (Chapter 4). It is critical for organists to understand that playing movements do not originate exclusively in the shoulder joint, but rather involve movement of the shoulder blades and the sternoclavicular joint as well. This mobility, or humero-scapular rhythm, must be understood, properly mapped, and claimed in order to reach to upper keyboards freely and fluently.

Balance and Movement on the Rockers

Find your rockers, sit bones, ischial tuberosities. Whatever you call them, or however you choose to think of them, find them! Organists must learn to sit on, balance on, and move on these two bony parts of the pelvis. Sit on the bench and rock, side to side, back to front. Tilt your pelvis backwards and forwards. Rock, tilt, explore. Go too far in virtually every direction, then return to what seems like a place of balance. Finding, mapping, and balancing on the rockers is critical for an organist. There is no other proper and comfortable way of sitting and moving on an organ bench.

On a personal note, when I first began my period of recovery from pain many years ago, I was concerned only with my hands and wrists. That's where the pain was. When Barbara Conable pointed out to me that I was sitting on the bench improperly, my internal and unspoken reaction was, "So what?" In fact, I was sitting on my tailbone. Go ahead and try that. Sit back on your tailbone. Notice that your lower back is rounded. Notice that your head is now pulled forward and down. Notice also the tension in your neck and upper back. Move your hands to a keyboard and notice that you feel like you are having to reach out. While still in this position, play a simple piece or hymn using the pedals. You will probably feel very uncomfortable, and if you practiced in this position for very long, you would begin to hurt. In fact, you might eventually injure yourself. Now, gently ease back up and onto your rockers. Notice that your spine begins to feel longer and more flexible. Your head will return to its proper place of balance on top of the spine. Movement of the legs, arms, and hands will now be easy and free.

Movement at the Hip Joint

In order to balance properly on the rockers and move the legs freely, organists must have a very clear understanding of the hip joint, and practice moving from that joint while seated on the bench. First, read again that portion of this book devoted to mapping the hip joint (Chapter 3). Then sit on the bench. Check the balance of the head on the spine. Confirm that you are balanced on the rockers. Then begin to move from the hip joints, observing kinesthetically the movement available to you. First singly, then together, extend your legs outward to the left and right as far as you can reach. Balance yourself by placing your hands on the bench or by grasping the ends of the keyboard. Notice what happens at the rockers and through the torso to facilitate this. Now move your right foot to the lower part of the pedalboard, then move your left foot up to the upper part of the pedalboard. Extend, reach, move. This kind

of experimentation will quickly lead to a clearer understanding of how the hip joint can be used more freely while playing the organ. This freedom of movement at the hip joint must be discovered and then practiced.

Use of the Muscles of the Groin, Upper Leg, and Buttocks

The muscles of the upper leg, buttocks, and groin must be actively involved in movements of the hip joints, legs, and feet. As you discover your place of balance on your rockers, and as you explore and cultivate the mobility you have at the hip joint, become aware of the muscles in the groin, upper legs, and buttocks. If you are involved in sports, yoga, running, walking, or stretching, you probably already have a kinesthetic awareness of these muscles. Otherwise you must again explore. I have found that getting off the bench and squatting on the floor puts me in touch immediately with these muscles. If you are unable to assume a squatting position, sit on a low bench or the edge of a chair and lean forward with your elbows on your knees. Be sure you are bending forward at your hip joints, and not from your waist. Move from side to side. Lean forward and lift your butt off the chair. These movements will involve the very muscles you need to be aware of as you play the organ. Take this awareness to the organ bench and experiment with it. There should be a fluid ripple of work from one set of muscles to another as you move on the bench.

If you identify your body through tension, that is, if you are aware of these muscles only because they are chronically tightened, you must first learn to release this chronic tension. Using muscles that are in a chronic state of tension or overwork will feel very different from using muscles that are supple and fluid. Tensed muscles inhibit free movement while playing and cause an unpleasant sensation of overwork. These organ-playing muscles must be supple and free if your playing is to be comfortable. Any excessive or chronic tension in these muscles must be replaced with the kinesthetic awareness of the muscles and their proper use.

Movement of the Ankle Joint

Organists should read again the portion of this book where the mapping of the ankle joint is discussed (Chapter 3). Once the map of the ankle joint is clear, movements of this joint should be practiced, both away from and at the organ. Again, sit on the organ bench and begin moving the ankle in all directions. Move first as though you were opening and closing a swell box (flexion and extension). Then work the ankle through its entire range of motion from side to side. Take these movements to the pedalboard and begin playing. Become aware, also, of the three playing surfaces available on the foot: the heel, the ball of the foot behind the big toe, and the ball of the foot behind the little toe.

❧

TECHNIQUE ISSUES AND GESTURES

Pedal Techniques

It is commonly accepted now that organists have two basic pedal techniques available to them: 1) toe-heel technique, used in repertoire from about 1800 on, and 2) all-toe technique for repertoire before 1800. All-toe technique implies a non-legato touch, and the use of alternate toes or the same foot moving laterally. Please note that this is not a discussion of technique or performance practice as such, but rather two different ways of moving. However you choose to play the pedals, you need to know how to move.

If you are using a toe-heel technique you must be sitting in a position on the bench that enables your heels to contact the pedals without effort. You must not feel that you are having to reach or push down with your heels, as this will distort your position of balance. A toe-heel technique will involve significant movement at the ankle joint. Read again the chapter in this book that discusses the ankle. Be sure you have clearly mapped your ankle joint and know how it moves. When you use an all-toe technique, you will need the bench to be higher. Your heels should be somewhat high and out of the way. It is also crucial to notice that with the all-toe technique there is much more movement from the hip joint, more movement of the whole leg, and much less movement at the ankle.

Position of the Bench

There are two measurements to consider for choosing your bench position: the height and its distance forward or back from the console. Your choice of pedal technique and the length of your lower leg will dictate the height of the bench. It is your physical relationship to the manuals, however, that should be the primary factor in determining the distance of the bench from the console. Pick the primary keyboard (usually the Great) and position yourself so that you have freedom to rock both forward and back on the bench. Most organists sit too close, and as a result are inhibited in their ability to move their arms freely. This in turn can cause tension in the back, chest, and upper limbs.

Knees Together or Not?

Many modern method books advocate a pedal technique which requires that the knees be kept together while playing the pedals. The logic behind this approach is appealing; however, a clear and thorough mapping of the body will ultimately lead to a pedal technique which allows the knees to move apart, sometimes rather far apart. Let's explore the logic of each approach.

1) Knees together. If the knees are kept together they provide a point of reference for measuring certain intervals. The fifth, C to G, will feel essentially the same as the fifth, A to E. The distances don't change, and if the knees are kept together, the intervals can be measured accurately and predictably.

2) Knees apart. Keep in mind that the human body was made to move. Holding the knees together while playing inhibits free movement, not only of the hip joints, but of the feet, hips, spine, neck, head, arms, and hands as well. Maintaining freedom of movement must override any pedagogical notion that measuring intervals with the knees together is desirable or even necessary. As your kinesthetic sense develops, the body will learn to measure intervals very accurately, not from a fixed point (the locked knees), but from fluid points of reference. The knees-apart approach concerns itself with the distance each foot moves individually, not with the distance one foot is from the other. If your left foot is on C you will know kinesthetically how far you must move to play G. Most assuredly, as you

refine your body map and learn to move authentically at the organ, you will find yourself abandoning the idea that the knees should be kept together.

Organists move their feet in virtually all directions while playing the organ. It is important to understand from where movement originates. A common mapping problem for organists who keep their knees together has to do with the movement of the lower leg from side to side, as for example while moving the right foot from a C up to G. Many organists have this movement mapped as originating in the knee. In fact, this side-to-side movement of the lower leg originates in the hip. Try this: sit on the organ bench facing away from the keyboards. Swing your lower legs front to back. This movement involves the knee. Now, swing the lower legs from side to side. This is movement at the hip. It is crucial for organists to get this sorted out. Failing to understand this can cause unwanted tension in the entire lower body.

⁂

SPECIFIC BALANCE AND MOVEMENT CONCERNS

Both Hands and Feet at the Center of Their Keyboards

When both hands and feet are playing more or less at the center of the keyboard, the temptation is to keep the elbows too close to the torso. In most cases, this is the result of mismapping the shoulder joint. This results in a lack of freedom of movement, leading to unwanted tension and lack of balance. Playing the organ should feel very much like hugging or wrapping your arms and legs around a tree. The upper back should be wide and the arms need to be free to move both out and around. Remember that your shoulder joint faces to the side, not to the front, and that this joint floats with the shoulder blade, allowing for a great deal of mobility and freedom.

Hands and Feet Both at the Same End of Their Keyboards

When both hands and both feet are at the low end of the keyboard and pedalboard, the temptation is for the limbs to reach in that direction while keeping the torso strictly vertical and facing forward. As a result, the right arm and elbow compress against the right side of the torso, restricting free movement. Instead, when playing hands and feet at the low end, or high end, of the keyboard and pedalboard, the entire torso should face in that direction as the arms move out and around, and the legs extend from the hip joints. In other words, turn in the direction you are playing and rise up on the rockers. Don't simply continue facing forward. Keep in mind that in this position, as well as while facing forward, the upper arm should be allowed to move in front of the torso. This is part of the wrapping or hugging gesture mentioned earlier, and can only be accomplished if the shoulder joint is properly mapped.

Hands at Low End, Feet at High End, or the Reverse

This position—hands low and feet high, or hands high and feet low—presents another challenge. If the hands are playing in the upper part of the keyboard while the feet are playing in the lower range of the pedalboard, your weight must shift onto the right rocker. At the same time, your spine must lengthen, bend, and spiral, and you should feel as though you were about to stand up on your right leg.

Hands on Separate Keyboards, Left Hand in a Higher Range Than the Right

Organists (and pianists) often suffer from the notion that the fingers must align themselves as though they were extensions of the keys. If the fingers are aligned in a straight line with the keys and this alignment is maintained as the left hand moves to an upper range of the keyboard, the result is severe ulnar deviation. The elbow of the left arm will also compress against the left side of the torso, causing tension and lack of mobility. Instead, allow the arms to float out and around. The fingers will relate to the keys at more natural angles, and balance of the body will be maintained. As an illustration, imagine the windshield wipers of a car. The blade does not wipe in a horizontal plane across the windshield, but rather, in an arc which forms ever-changing angles. Take that illustration to the keyboard and experiment with it.

Continuous Motion and Follow-through

Music moves. In order to play freely and musically, organists must move also. When the body map is accurate, when the muscles are free and fluid, and when inhibitions are discarded, movement will be continuous, just as air moving into pipes is continuous and fluid. The body in continuous motion must not be held in a fixed position. Organists very often sit rigidly on the bench, facing forward as though driving a car. Watch any good musician move while playing or singing. There is continuous and free movement of the body. How do you know how to move, and in which direction? Move the way the music moves. Move as the musical lines move with your arm structure, your head, and your spine. Remember also that a place of balance is a place we move in and out of. Being in balance is like a consonant interval; moving momentarily out of balance is like a dissonant interval, which then resolves to consonance (balance) once more.

Another related concept organists often fail to grasp is that of follow-through. Imagine a tennis player hitting a ball. The racket does not stop moving as soon as the ball is hit. There is a follow-through gesture as the movement of the racket continues. This is true in virtually all sports activities, and should be true as well when playing a keyboard instrument. Imagine yourself playing an ascending solo line in the right hand. If movement is correct, the arm structure will lead that line upward. When the end of the musical line is reached there should be a f ollow-through gesture as the arm structure continues some movement in the direction the musical line was going. Now imagine playing a chord. What may seem like a simple musical gesture, when analyzed carefully, is actually a complicated and interwoven series of gestures involving movement. There will be downward movement, some lateral movement of the wrist, upward movement on the release of the chord, and movement involving the entire arm structure. The point to be made here is that there should be continuous movement, and that this continuous movement will involve a series of follow-through gestures. It is easier to remain in motion than to be continually stopping movement and starting it again. Careful observation and analysis of good playing will reveal thousands of examples of continuous motion and follow-through. Organists need to explore, observe, and learn these gestures if free and easy playing is to be accomplished.

Organists, Think Joints!

Organists more than anyone else need all of their joints, as well as whole-body awareness, while playing. Many organists sit on the bench stiffly, facing forward, afraid to move more than their hands and feet. They may wonder why they are uncomfortable, or even in pain. Organ playing requires a very accurate body map. It requires both a physical and mental awareness that movement while playing the organ is good. From the feet, through the legs, pelvis, spine, arm structure, hands, neck, and head—all parts of the body should contribute freely to organ playing.

CHAPTER 9: INJURIES AND RETRAINING

The first chapters of this book emphasized that injuries come from chronically tense movement. In them, I presented anatomical facts which can help pianists improve their body maps and the quality of their movement. In this chapter I recapitulate and expand some of the points made in earlier chapters of the book, but from a different point of view. First, I take a physical approach and describe the typical ways in which tense movement can lead to injury and offer brief descriptions of specific injuries. I then give reasons why movement retraining must be a part of any permanent cure and link the concept of retraining with the concept of Body Mapping. Finally, I describe some of the psychological obstacles faced by injured pianists.

֍

FOUR CAUSES OF INJURY

Co-contraction

Our arms and hands are moved by muscles. Muscles exert force only when they contract, so each muscle can exert force in only one direction. To move a body part in two directions requires two muscles or two sets of muscles, one to move it one way and one to move it the other way. When one muscle contracts, the opposing muscle must release and lengthen to permit movement. If this does not happen—that is, if the opposing muscle remains tense—then both muscles are con-tracting simultaneously, which is called *co-contraction*. Co-contraction inhibits movement and can cause injury.

Awkward Positions

A muscle attaches to the bone it moves by means of a tendon, and the tendon passes over a joint (or several joints). The relative position of the bones will influence the efficiency of the tendon in transmitting the muscular force to the part moved, especially in cases like the fingers where the tendon passes over several joints. Awkward or extreme positions of the wrist and hand stress these tendons, making movement more difficult and also weaker. The mid-range position of the wrist, with the wrist in approximately a straight line with the fore-arm, gives the greatest mechanical advantage to the fingers. Awkward positions make movement stressful and can cause injury.

Static Muscular Activity

Typically, when a muscle exerts force to move a body part, the muscle contracts and decreases in length as the part moves. When the part moves the other way, the muscle releases and lengthens. Thus, the muscle alternately gets shorter and longer. This kind of activity is called *dynamic*. But if the muscle exerts force without changing in length, the activity is called *static*. This is the type of activity used in isometric exercises. Static muscular activity is more stressful than dynamic activity. Dynamic activity permits circulation of the blood, whereas static muscular activity inhibits blood circulation, causing the muscle to become fatigued and making it prone to injury.

Excessive Force

Obviously, stress to the muscles, tendons, and other vulnerable structures varies according to the amount of force used: more force is more stressful than less force. But this does not make clear how damaging excessive force can be. According to some studies, doubling the force multiplies stress on the tendons not by two but by five. Depressing keys on the piano does not require much force; the standard touch weight for a well-regulated piano is only fifty grams, about the weight of ten U.S. five-cent pieces. It is easy for pianists to fall into the habit of using more force than needed, and because of the extremely high levels of repetition involved in piano playing, excessive force is potentially injurious.

In short, pianists' stress injuries are caused by:

1) co-contraction
2) awkward positions
3) static muscular activity
4) excessive force

These factors, alone or in combination, are the source of virtually all the pain and discomfort experienced by pianists.

Although stressful movements are the cause of injury, there are other factors that contribute to the body's resistance to injury and its ability to recover. A person's general health is one factor, physical fitness

is another. Rest is also important. A person who gets adequate rest will be more resistant. Another factor is age. The body's ability to resist injury lessens as we get older. This is why some pianists play for years without problems, and then later, in their thirties or forties, they develop an injury. They are not playing differently, but their body's ability to withstand the strain has lessened.

༄

HOW INJURY DEVELOPS

Power to move our fingers, hands, and arms comes from muscles, which are attached by tendons to the parts they move. Some tendons are quite long. For example, since the muscles that move the fingers are mostly in the back of the forearm, the tendons to the fingers extend through the wrist and hand. Tendons are like long, fibrous cords. They are made of collagen, they are not very elastic, and they are very strong. They slide back and forth as we move our arms and fingers, some by as much as two and a half inches. To facilitate the back-and-forth movement, tendons may be enclosed in sheaths for part or all of their length. These are the synovial sheaths, which secrete a fluid (synovial fluid) that acts as a lubricant. Circulation of blood in the tendons is limited, which means that if a tendon becomes injured, recovery is slow.

For pianists and others who engage in repetitive motion, the tendons are the weak link in the system, the structures especially prone to stress injury. Most stress injuries of the hand, wrist, arm, and shoulders involve the tendons. To be sure, muscles can also be injured, but they recover more quickly. The four causes of injury listed above are dangerous because they increase stress on the tendons.

Tendons become injured because of repeated tensing or from rubbing on nearby ligaments and bones. Subjected to constant stress, tendons may fray or tear apart, or become thickened and bumpy. The injured area may calcify. The tendon sheath is also vulnerable; it may produce excess fluid, causing swelling. The tendon may become "locked" in the sheath and move jerkily; the sheath may become inflamed and press on the tendon. Inflammation and swelling in the restricted space of the carpal tunnel can put pressure on the median nerve, leading to the tingling and numbness of the thumb and second finger which often indicate carpal tunnel syndrome. All this starts to sound like a catalogue of medieval tortures, and for pianists who have been injured it might as well be just that. Symptoms include aching, tenderness, tingling, soreness—in short, pain. The pain can be so severe as to prevent not only piano playing but everyday actions as well. One pianist (now fully recovered and playing beautifully) says that when suffering from acute tendonitis the mere lifting of a paperback book was excruciating.

How does it come about that a good pianist may play in a way that stresses the body? I think there are two principal reasons. First, most people's technique is not deliberately chosen. That is, the person does not analyze the movements needed to play a passage and practice those movements. Instead, the person just finds a way, by hook or crook and trial and error, to get to the right notes. With constant repetition the movements become

habits. Sometimes, movements acquired this way will be efficient. But there is no guarantee. Our bodies can become used to inefficient movements as well as efficient ones, and when we are used to them, the inefficient ones feel "normal." The movements that can cause injury do not necessarily feel bad or painful. Indeed, they are not dangerous in non-repetitive tasks. They are dangerous for pianists because piano playing is extremely repetitive.

The second way in which people come to move stressfully is that they are taught stressful movements. No teacher would knowingly teach harmful movements. But too few teachers understand the principles of efficient movement, and some ways of moving that are dangerous to our health are firmly established in traditional pedagogy. "Wrist octaves," for example, which are still recommended by some pianists and teachers, cannot be performed at the required level of repetition without danger because, as typically taught and practiced, they involve static muscular activity, co-contraction, and excessive force.

⁓

TENDONITIS

Most pianists' injuries are injuries to the tendons of the arm and hand—that is, some form of tendonitis. Names and spellings vary. "Tendonitis" and "tendinitis" are equivalent; "tenosynovitis" refers to injuries involving the synovial sheath that surrounds the tendon. "De Quervain's disease" affects tendons of the thumb. "Lateral epicondylitis" or "tennis elbow" affects tendons on the outside of the elbow, "medial epicondylitis" or "golfer's elbow" affects tendons on the inside of the elbow. "Ganglion cysts" are disorders of the tendon sheaths. There are also injuries to the tendons in the shoulder. Shoulder injuries may affect the tendons in the rotator cuff or the bursa, which is the cushion underlying the tendon and protecting it. Injuries to the bursa are called "bursitis." Injuries to the tendons receive different names depending on the specific structure that is affected. All these problems can occur in pianists, though few pianists suffer from all at once (thank goodness!). All of them are use-related: they result from the pianist's way of using the arm and hand. In almost all cases they will heal if the pianist adopts a better use. On the other hand, if a pianist persists in moving with tension, they can lead to permanent damage.

Why should pianists (and other people who use their hands in repetitive tasks) be subject to tendon injuries? The answer is obvious the moment we look at the array of muscles that move the hand and fingers.

Almost all pianists are familiar with exercises designed to "strengthen the fingers." But few pianists seem to know that the muscles that move the fingers are not in the fingers. There are no muscles in the fingers. The fingers are moved partly by muscles in the hand, but most of the work is done by muscles in the forearm. These muscles do not attach directly to the different joints of the fingers, they attach by means of long tendons. There are separate muscles for the various joints of the different fingers, each with its own tendon. There are some twenty-four tendons attaching to different parts of the hand and fingers—nine extensor tendons to the thumb and fingers, one abductor tendon to the thumb, two extensor tendons to the hand, three flexor tendons to the hand, and nine flexor tendons to the fingers and thumb. In an anatomical drawing the tendons look like strands of spaghetti arranged neatly parallel by a fastidious cook. Tendon problems often arise near joints where the tendons rub on ligaments or bones, and they also result from repeated tensing of the muscle-tendon unit. Every pianist should examine an illustration of the muscles and tendons of the arm and hand (see page 106). The picture gives a vivid sense of the length of the tendons and their vulnerability to various kinds of misuse. Looking at an illustration makes clear why awkward positions, excessive force, co-contraction, and static muscular tension will put extra stress on the tendons. The same information can become the basis of an improved body map and a better quality of movement. Pianists and teachers with this knowledge will be better able to prevent or recover from injury, and better able to help their students.

✌

CARPAL TUNNEL SYNDROME

The carpal tunnel is a narrow space formed by the small bones of the wrist and the ligament called the flexor retinaculum. You can locate it this way: place your left index finger in the center of your right palm, then move the finger about two inches down your palm toward your arm, stopping when your finger approaches the edge of the fleshy part of your hand. Your finger now lies directly over the carpal tunnel. The carpal tunnel is formed by the small bones of the wrist which combine to make a U-shaped depression with bones on the bottom and sides. The flexor retinaculum ligament stretches over the top of the U to create a tunnel. The space in the tunnel is small—about as big as the end of your thumb.

Nine flexor tendons, two to each finger and one to the thumb, pass through the carpal tunnel. The space is so narrow that some of the tendons are stacked on top of each other to form two layers, instead of running side by side the way they do outside the tunnel. The tendons in the tunnel are enclosed in sheaths. The median nerve also passes through the carpal tunnel. The median nerve supplies most of the palm, the thumb, fingers 2 and 3, and part of finger 4.

The carpal tunnel is a nifty structure, well-designed to do its job of providing a space for the tendons. It is vulnerable because it is small. Like a tightly packed suitcase, it has no space for any additional items. If the tendons or their sheaths are subject to stressful movement, they may become inflamed and swollen. This is a problem because any swelling by the tendons or their sheaths within the tunnel puts pressure on the other tendons, and also on the median nerve. The nerve may become compressed. The result is carpal tunnel syndrome: pain in the wrist, and pain or tingling or numbness in the hand, particularly on the thumb side of the hand. Sometimes the hand feels weak or clumsy. The symptoms may be worst at night.

Carpal tunnel syndrome is usually caused by movements that put repetitive stress on the tendons in the carpal tunnel. Examples of dangerous movements include repetitive forceful flexing of the wrist, as in "wrist octaves." "Dropping the wrist" is also dangerous (think of the wrist supports that are increasingly common among computer users), as is thumb-oriented movement, particularly if it is accompanied by tightness across the wrist, as when a person moves the wrist as a hinge (see the section on the wrist and hand).

Surgical treatment for carpal tunnel syndrome involves cutting the flexor retinaculum to create more space for the tendons and the median nerve. This surgery may produce immediate relief, but unfortunately, the relief is often temporary. If the person continues to move in a stressful manner, symptoms are likely to return. The best permanent cure is movement retraining, which makes surgery unnecessary.

Sometimes symptoms of carpal tunnel syndrome do not come from misuse of the hand and forearm but from misuse of the upper arm. If a person habitually uses the upper arm in a way that causes the collarbone to put pressure on the median nerve where it passes under the collarbone, the symptoms may be the same as if pressure were placed on the median nerve in the carpal tunnel. It is, after all, the same nerve. When the problem originates in the upper arm it is called "thoracic outlet syndrome."

❧

DYSTONIA

Dystonia is distinct from injuries like tendonitis that affect muscles and tendons. In dystonia the brain's capacity to control movement is impaired. Muscles may tighten involuntarily, producing awkward, jerky movements. Hands or fingers may fail to respond to conscious commands, or respond in unintended ways. Fingers may clench involuntarily instead of touching the intended key. The condition may not be painful, but the emotional stress and frustration endured by musicians suffering from dystonia is immense. Dystonia has ended the careers of some famous and wonderful musicians.

Dystonia can affect any part of the body, and it takes many forms. Some dystonias are devastating conditions that affect large areas of the body, distort posture and speech, and make driving, walking, talking, or eating difficult or impossible. Some dystonias seem to be congenital, perhaps genetic. The cause of these conditions is not well understood, nor is there any reliable cure.

Other forms of dystonia are not congenital but appear later in life. Acquired dystonia often affects only a specific part of the body, perhaps just one finger, which may uncontrollably clench or freeze or shoot out to the side. Dystonia of this sort is called "focal dystonia" and it is the sort that most often occurs in pianists. Focal dystonia usually affects parts of the body that are subject to constant use in an activity like writing or piano playing. Sometimes the affected part, a finger, for example, responds normally in other activities and becomes uncontrollable only in the context of the specific activity of writing or piano playing.

The cause of focal dystonia is not precisely known. No one, I believe, is yet in a position to state the necessary and sufficient conditions for the development of focal dystonia, nor to say exactly what neurological events occur or fail to occur when a pianist loses control of her fingers. Moreover, there is no medical cure for dystonia—none, that is, that counts as a cure in the way penicillin is a cure for strep infection, where the cure is reliable, we know why it works, and we can explain those cases when it doesn't work. In

the sense of "cure" according to which a doctor administers the cure and the patient is well again, there is no cure for dystonia.

Nevertheless, the situation is not hopeless for pianists or other musicians with focal dystonia. There are many musicians who have recovered from dystonia and returned to full playing. There may be no medical cure for dystonia, but there are movement therapies that have been consistently successful in cases of musicians' focal dystonia. The successful therapies start from an empirically observed connection between dystonia and certain patterns of movement. When a person changes those patterns, the condition can eventually resolve. Some forms of movement retraining are more effective than others. Concentrating on technique alone is not always effective; there are pianists who have undertaken to cure their dystonia by rebuilding their technique but have made little progress after lengthy (and expensive) training. An approach that emphasizes overall coordination of the whole body is generally more successful than concentrating on training just the hand and fingers. Admittedly, this is a delicate process. It requires consistency, vigilant attention, time, and collaboration with a knowledgeable teacher. No one knows for certain whether this approach will help all musicians with dystonia, but it has been consistently successful with those who have followed it. One thing that seems clear is that developing a sense of embodiment, training the kinesthetic sense, acquiring an accurate and adequate body map, constantly relating the part to the whole—the recurrent themes, in short, of this book—are vital in the resolution of dystonia.

Why movement retraining is effective in cases of dystonia is a matter for speculation. It is tempting to imagine that what happens is a reeducation of the brain-hand relationship. Perhaps it is a matter of creating new neural pathways that will reliably transmit the commands from the brain to the fingers and send information back from the fingers to the brain. These are topics of active research for neurophysiologists. For musicians, the final answer on those questions is less important than the knowledge that recovery from dystonia is possible.

ↄ

CURE OF INJURY

The good news about injury is that we can be cured. Our bodies have an amazing capacity to repair themselves, and injuries will heal, provided that they have not been allowed to progress to the point of permanent damage. Even the tendons, despite their limited blood supply, will recover in time. In the acute phase of an injury, treatment may involve rest, anti-inflammatories to reduce inflammation and swelling, and massage, which can stimulate circulation (producing some of the benefits of exercise without actually having to work the injured structure). What these "treatments" really do is to provide conditions in which the body's own healing powers can do their job.

All this is marvelous, but far too often the cure is only temporary because the person returns to the same activity as before and performs it in the same stressful way, causing reinjury. A permanent cure requires *identifying and removing the cause* of the injury. Now, we know that piano playing need not be injurious, since many people, including

some fabulous virtuosos, do it without ever injuring themselves. Therefore, the fact of someone being injured does not prove that piano playing is dangerous in itself. What it does prove is that there was something in the technique that was stressful, something that with constant repetition over years of playing resulted in injury. The person must learn to play the piano using non-stressful movements to perform the tasks that were formerly performed with stressful movements. In short, a permanent cure for pianists' injuries requires *movement retraining*.

For the pianist who recognizes all this, the information in this book is invaluable. Body Mapping is an extraordinarily powerful tool in retraining. More strongly, developing an accurate and adequate body map is at bottom *one and the same as* movement retraining. The habits of movement— co-contraction, awkward positions, static muscular activity, and excessive force—that produce physical symptoms can all be seen as mapping errors. If I mismap the rotation of my forearm and use my arm chronically in a thumb-oriented way, the tension in the superficial muscles of my forearm leads to— indeed it *amounts to*—one or more of the physical causes of injury: co-contraction, awkward positions, static muscular activity, or excessive force. If I mismap the motion needed to execute a passage, the same thing may happen: the mismapping causes me to move—or *amounts to* my moving—in a way that may include one of the causes of injury.

A pianist who develops an improved body map and a vivid kinesthetic sense can move with awareness, in accord with the structure, freely and easily doing things that were formerly tense and difficult. As sensitivity and awareness grow, the playing improves and injury can heal because the pianist has removed its cause.

❧
WHY MANY PIANISTS DO NOT RECOVER

Saying that to cure an injury we must remove its cause sounds too obvious to require emphasis, but in fact movement retraining, which is the way to accomplish this, very often does not happen. There are several reasons why injured pianists often do not get the retraining that would cure their injuries.

Very often, people don't understand the need for retraining or believe in the possibility of moving differently to play the piano. After all, they play the piano the way they always have done, the way they were taught to play. Consequently, when first injured they rarely look for someone to analyze their technique, identify the problem, and find a solution. Instead they resort to transparently poor strategies like denial, wishful thinking, or "toughing it out." They say, "I'll rest over the weekend and it will be better on Monday," or "I guess I just overdid it, I'll take it easy for a while." Sometimes the first symptoms are even welcomed, and people say, "I must really be making progress in my practicing, I can feel it in my arms" (the "no pain, no gain" fallacy). Or else, misled by discussions in the literature, they say, "I just tried to do too much without proper warm-up; I'll be careful always to warm up from now on," or "I guess I need to exercise and develop strength in my fingers." As the injury persists, they become desperate. They

go to doctors, physical therapists, chiropractors, accupuncturists, nutritionists, massage therapists—anyone at all. Some of these professionals can help, especially in treating the acute condition, but their help is limited and often temporary. They are not trained to do what is really necessary, namely to teach the person how to play the piano without danger of reinjury.

Piano periodicals and books on technique are not generally very helpful to the injured pianist. Few discussions of pianists' injuries emphasize movement retraining, and the strategies they do recommend are not especially effective, either for avoiding or for curing injury. These include "building endurance," "developing strength," taking frequent breaks, warming up, "pacing oneself," and the like. In themselves, I have no quarrel with any of these suggestions; all are good things to do, and they may contribute to our ability to resist injury. But they are not the full answer; someone can do all of them and still be injured. For example, suppose my way of playing octaves involves forcefully flexing my wrist. There are anatomical reasons why repeated forceful flexion of the wrist is dangerous; it is, in fact, one of the common causes of carpal tunnel syndrome. Therefore, if that is how I play octaves I am risking injury. Even if I take breaks, warm up before practicing, and so on, it will still be true that with every octave I play I will be stressing the tendons in my wrist. If I use stressful movements to play octaves, then telling me to avoid injury by warming up before practicing the Sixth Hungarian Rhapsody is like telling a smoker to take some deep breaths before lighting up in order to avoid lung cancer. Warming up and deep breathing are great, but they don't remove the cause of the problem. Just as lung cancer is caused by smoking, not by failure to do lung exercises, so pianists' injuries are caused by tense movement, not by failure to warm up, take breaks, and so on.

Becoming injured can be emotionally devastating for a pianist. If a person's thoughts, aspirations, and, perhaps, very livelihood center around the piano, then to be unable to play one's best, unable to play without pain, perhaps unable to play at all, is a dreadful experience. Injured pianists often become deeply depressed and discouraged. The injury can become a stigma and the injured pianist feels isolated, rejected, inadequate, and humiliated. Depression and a sense of hopelessness can themselves be obstacles to recovery. An injured pianist desperately needs emotional support and understanding from friends, relatives, colleagues, and teachers.

Unfortunately, many colleagues and teachers, though well-intentioned and sympathetic, can offer only limited help. Typically, they offer moral support, which is essential, but few have a clear understanding of the causes of injury or the conditions for recovery; few have the information they need to prevent injury in their students or show an injured pianists how to recover. What I described a few paragraphs back as "transparently poor strategies" are the ones most often invoked by teachers and pianists at all levels. This is understandable; after all, the required information is not part of most music curricula, pedagogy classes, or conservatory programs. On the assumption, natural enough but usually mistaken, that the problem is a medical problem, not a movement problem, teachers and colleagues may send the injured pianist

for medical treatment or therapy. Such treatment rarely produces a complete, permanent cure, so teachers and colleagues feel helpless, frustrated, and anguished along with the injured pianist. The general problem will be solved only when sound information is part of every pianist's training. When teachers have the information and students, from the very beginning, are taught according to the principles offered here, pianists' injuries will no longer occur.

For an injured pianist, learning to move safely at the piano will require abandoning old physical habits and replacing them with new ones. I have described how to do that. The approach I have presented does work, but it takes time and application, and the project of abandoning old ways may seem daunting at first. But there is a deeper problem as well: the old ways may be embedded not just in our bodies but in our minds. Suppose I have been injured by my way of playing octaves. Suppose further, though, that I was taught to play octaves by a teacher whom I deeply admire. When I learn that my way of playing octaves has caused my injury, it may cause me to question or modify my opinion of my former teacher. It may lead me to rethink many aspects of my own teaching and playing. I may be obliged to conclude that things I formerly believed sincerely were not actually the best. *In short, movement retraining forces me to examine myself and my relationship with the piano, and I must be prepared to question and change my attitudes and beliefs.* Even if the results make the effort worthwhile, the process is not easy.

Another obstacle is the sports analogy. In our sports-oriented society, comparisons with sports are everywhere and they can be very harmful. All too often, piano students are encouraged to think of themselves as if they were engaged in a competitive sport. They are told they need to develop strength and endurance. I recently received some promotional material touting some finger weights that are "guaranteed" to strengthen pianists' muscles and increase endurance. That there is a market for such products shows the influence of the mindless analogy with sports that pervades a lot of pedagogical writing and thinking. (Has no one heard of Robert Schumann?) In fact, playing the piano is not very much like an endurance sport, and building a technique is not a matter of building muscles. The amount of physical strength required to play the piano is very little, and endurance is not an issue if one is moving efficiently. Playing the piano is a complex physical skill which involves the whole mind and body and spirit. It requires that we move rapidly and efficiently, but it is not a matter of strength or endurance.

The sports analogy infects our ways of dealing with injury; we may say "no pain, no gain" when our arms are sore, and continue practicing in the same way. If our hands feel weak—a frequent symptom of injury—we think the answer is to do strengthening exercises. In fact this may only make the problem worse. If a structure is injured, working it harder will not promote healing. Some (very few) comparisons with sports may be useful, but for the most part the sports analogy is misleading and harmful.

Throughout this book I have advocated movement retraining based on developing an adequate and accurate body map as the way to avoid or cure injury. But we should always remember that injury, serious as it is, is not the most compelling reason for improving the quality of our movement. The most compelling reason is this: *we play better if we move efficiently*. Many pianists have retrained after injury because it was the only way they could play at all, and found that they could play better than before. Others have retrained without being injured and found the same thing: they can play better, play with greater ease, play more difficult repertoire, and overcome technical problems that formerly seemed hopeless. Improving the quality of our movement at the piano is not only the way to cure or avoid injury, it is the best way to achieve our artistic goals.

CONCLUSION

I hope that reading this book has already made a difference in your playing—that you have found some fact, some bit of information that you could incorporate into your movement at the piano and achieve a better result. If so, you have already discovered for yourself how an improved body map can support and enable your playing. That experience will do more than any words of mine to convince you of the power of the information offered here. What I can tell you, however, is that what you have so far is just the beginning, a mere taste. As you develop greater kinesthetic sensitivity and refine your body map, you will make further progress.

I urge you to take an active, experimental, questioning approach. "Is my upper arm truly free? What happens if I allow it to participate?" "How can my spine adjust to help me play this passage?" "Can I be better grounded on the bench and feel support up through the core?" Try novel ways of moving and reject what doesn't work. Question authority and tradition. Do not take for granted that the motions you have been using—the ones you were taught or the ones taken for granted by pedagogues—are always the best solutions. Allow your body to move as needed to support your playing. You won't injure yourself if you move with knowledge and awareness of your structure. Instead, you will learn to find better solutions to technical and expressive problems. You will let the music, together with your kinesthetic sense, guide you to the motions that get the result you want.

You will discover that there is no end, no limit to the progress you can make, so long as you bear in mind that improving your playing and improving your movement are one and the same. We don't get better by repeating prescribed motions over and over, we get better by changing our motions to find the ones that get a better result.

Artur Rubinstein, in his eighties, is reported to have said that he was finally beginning to learn to play the piano. The remark might be taken as a joke, since he had been a world-famous pianist for sixty years. But I believe that he was perfectly sincere and that his comment attests to the freshness, the love of life, the welcoming of new experiences that characterized him—famously—throughout his life. We can adopt the same attitude. Playing the piano is complex, demanding, subtle; at times it can be frustrating or baffling. But it is also deeply rewarding and a source of ongoing personal growth. Whatever our age or level of skill, we can derive endless satisfaction from it if we approach it in the spirit I am advocating, armed with the information in this book. I wish you a lifetime of happiness and fulfillment in your piano playing.

℘

SUGGESTIONS FOR FURTHER READING OR REFERENCE

Atlas of Human Anatomy, by Frank H. Netter, M.D.
East Hanover, NJ: Novartis, Second Edition, 1997.

Human Structure, by Matt Cartmill, William L. Hylander
and James Shaffland. Cambridge, MA: Harvard University
Press, 1987.

Surface Anatomy, by James S.P. Lumley. London: Churchill
Livingstone, 1996.

Anatomy of Movement, by Blandine Calais-Germain.
Seattle: Eastland Press, 1993.

*Cumulative Trauma Disorders: A Manual for Musculoskeletal
Diseases of the Upper Limbs,* Vern Putz-Anderson, ed.
Cincinnati: Taylor & Francis, 1988.

The Hand, by Frank R. Wilson. New York: Pantheon Books, 1998.

How to Learn the Alexander Technique, by Barbara Conable.
Columbus, OH: Andover Press, Third Edition, 1995.

*Indirect Procedures: A Musician's Guide to the Alexander
Technique,* by Pedro de Alcantara. Oxford: Oxford
University Press, 1997.

~

THE AUTHORS

Thomas Mark teaches piano and Body Mapping in Portland, Oregon, and offers the course "What Every Pianist Needs to Know about the Body" throughout the United States and Canada. His website is www.pianomap.com.

Roberta Gary is Professor of Organ and Head of the Keyboard Division at the College-Conservatory of Music of the University of Cincinnati.

Thom Miles is Director of Music at Isaac M. Wise Temple and Assistant Organist at Christ Church Cathedral, Cincinnati, and a teacher of Suzuki piano.

Barbara Conable is founder of Andover Educators, a network of teachers saving, securing, and enhancing musical careers with accurate information about the body in movement (www.bodymap.org). She is author of three books about movement for musicians. She lives in Portland, Oregon, where she continues to develop the theory and practice of Body Mapping. She is adjunct faculty at Portland State University in the Coordinate Movement Program for Pianists (www.pianotechnique.org).